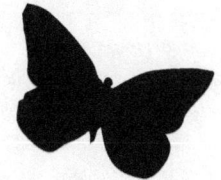

Single with Breast Cancer– My journey

by

Bruna Verna

authorHOUSE®

AuthorHouse™
1663 Liberty Drive, Suite 200
Bloomington, IN 47403
www.authorhouse.com
Phone: 1-800-839-8640

This book is a work of non-fiction. Unless otherwise noted, the author and the publisher make no explicit guarantees as to the accuracy of the information contained in this book and in some cases, names of people and places have been altered to protect their privacy.

First published by AuthorHouse   1/14/2008

ISBN: 978-1-4343-5220-0 (sc)
ISBN: 978-1-4343-5964-3 (hc)

Library of Congress Control Number: 2007909733

Printed in the United States of America
Bloomington, Indiana

This book is printed on acid-free paper.

A special thanks to Marybeth Zack.

Marybeth had the spirit that got me through many tough days.

Marybeth was my spinning instructor. She was an example for me while going through breast cancer. Leading spinning classes several times a week – she was the one that would push me to my limit while she was undergoing cancer treatments and chemo therapy. She allowed me to attend the most challenging workouts I have ever had in all of my life...and love every one of them.

She never quit and had a following that respected her in a way many will never see.

Marybeth is a spirit that made all of us believe we are not quitters.

You could not be in Marybeth's presence without being changed in some way.

Marybeth,

I met you at the most appropriate time in my life and I take you as a gift from God.

You will be remembered always

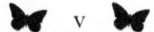 v

Preface

I knew on my journey with breast cancer I would overcome this disease and it would just be another bump in the road. It was my detour as I was continuing on a path I should not be on. All I have ever asked of God was to keep my children safe, happy and healthy and to be sure he did not take me away from my children too soon. God and I would know when the children no longer needed me in life and this was not that time.

I took Breast Cancer for what it was. 1 needed to get off this crazy path I continued to go on. My job was endless. I choose to be a workaholic thinking this would bring things I longed for in life and never got. I had less time with my family and friends. I had a niece that attended college in Newport, Rhode Island. This is only a two hour ride for me. My brother and his family live in Tampa, Florida. This was his daughter and I owed it to him as well as myself to find a closeness with Jess. I wanted to see her and form a close relationship as this was a beautiful opportunity for us. I kept putting off weekend visits because I had so much work to do. Four years went by and shame on me for letting this opportunity slide.

I was too busy to sit still with my own children. There was no reason for me not to make the time to go out to dinner often with them and keep up with their lives. I couldn't find the time to do this either. I worked evenings and weekends. Shame on me.

Breast Cancer came along and smacked me right between the eyes. God was making his statement and it was loud and clear to me this time. 1 was given the chance to reevaluate my life and start living it. I was given the chance to take hold of what I really wanted in this lifetime and make it happen. There is no good time and no reason to put things off. The right time, enough money and on and on will never happen. You are the holder of that key. You make it happen. However it needs to be you make your desires come into your life. You focus and figure out a way. There is always a way if you want something enough. If the dream is not worth you making it happen then you didn't want it enough. Let it go and make what you want happen. This is one life, one chance and no one should leave this show with a desire or to utter "I wish I did" - "I wish I could."

I would come to find out while being on this new path that I will make time to be with family and friends. I would figure out a way to make my dreams come true. All I had to do was listen and God would give me the way. When I would take someone's phone number and tell them I will call them - I will. I would appreciate the time with my children so much more. I would bring a pup I so desire for years into my life and he would bring the family closer than I had ever had it.

I was too busy to listen to what God was trying to tell me for years. I was not able to give it all up to God and felt I needed to control my life to make things happen myself. How foolish was I? Did I really think anything could happen without God's help? I was one of God's very stubborn children and God needed to sit me still and put just enough fear in my life to listen to him. To be thankful for what I have and not feel a need for what I don't have. I stopped dead in my tracks and everyday I am thankful, everyday I ask God's advice and I listen to God

I am blessed.

Dedication

I dedicate this book to my three children. Without them I would have never survived my struggles in life. They are the vision every morning to be all I can be in this lifetime. They are the reason I am writing these pages. They are my miracles in life and God's promise to me that nothing could ever take me unless they no longer need me in life.

Tony for his vision of truth. I am so proud of the man he has become. Not being afraid to show his sensitive side and not giving into the BS in this world. For keeping his own ground and doing what he believes and feels right or not doing it at all. I am proud when I look at Tony as a man and I notice how very handsome he is. His love has sustained me in many struggles in my life.

Christina for being sweet and honest and doing what she believes in. I am so proud of the beautiful young woman she has turned into. Her struggles to become what fits and feels right for her makes me believe she can live no other way than the right way for her in life. Continuing on this path she will get to where she is supposed to be. Her love has sustained me in many struggles in my life.

Erica for her spirit . I am so very proud of my sensitive and somewhat insecure at the moment daughter but a powerhouse of faith. I see myself in Erica and I believe once she has set out in life on her own and apart from my home she will become an incredibly successful woman. Her focus is so strong and there is no other way but to be what she was destined to be. Her honesty is beyond that of anyone I have ever met, including myself. Her faith will never alter in her life, and I believe this will keep her on the path she was meant to be in life. God gave her beauty she does not yet know she has. Her love has sustained me in many struggles in my life.

Tony, Chris, and Erica, I love you more than life itself. Thank you for listening to the meaningful things I have taught you in life. I am proud when I see how you have chosen to live out your lives.

I want to thank my children, Tony, Christina, and Erica for being the light in my life. For keeping me focused on what is important to me. For giving me the will to survive life and all its drama. The way I see it, the world is a Cirque de Sole. We are just a speck observing called the audience. There is so much going on onstage. The color, the talent—and it feels you are being pulled in all directions. It is so hard to stay focused on one thing, your path, your journey in life. It is so hard to stay centered when there is so much going on around you constantly. It seems to shut God out at times with all the distractions. Tony, Christina, and Erica always bring me back to that center space where God exists. I am thankful and so grateful.

I want to thank my younger brother Cam and his wife Marilyn. If it were not for them, I would never have gotten to where I am today. They were both there for me through my divorce, which broke me in every way possible in life. They held my hand, picked me back up, and taught me to stand tall once again. If I had not had this support at this time in my life, I believe I would not have stood a chance to fight breast cancer. It is all in your will, and my will was not allowed to be broken thanks to my brother and his wife. Marilyn has always been a sister to me. I could never have thought of her as just a sister-in-law. I thank them for showing me what family really is. I wish we did not have the geographical distance between us, but I am thankful and grateful for them in my life.

I want to thank everyone that I have been able to hold dear to me in life. When you go through a time in life as I did with breast cancer, it allows you to notice. You see things very clearly. You realize so much at that humble time. I am thankful and grateful for the people I can call friends and family today. The people that never left me alone . . . ever.

I want to thank God for the experience of this, for without it I would not know who I was, who I can become, and who is so dear in my life. I am also thankful and grateful for my special gift, Bailey.

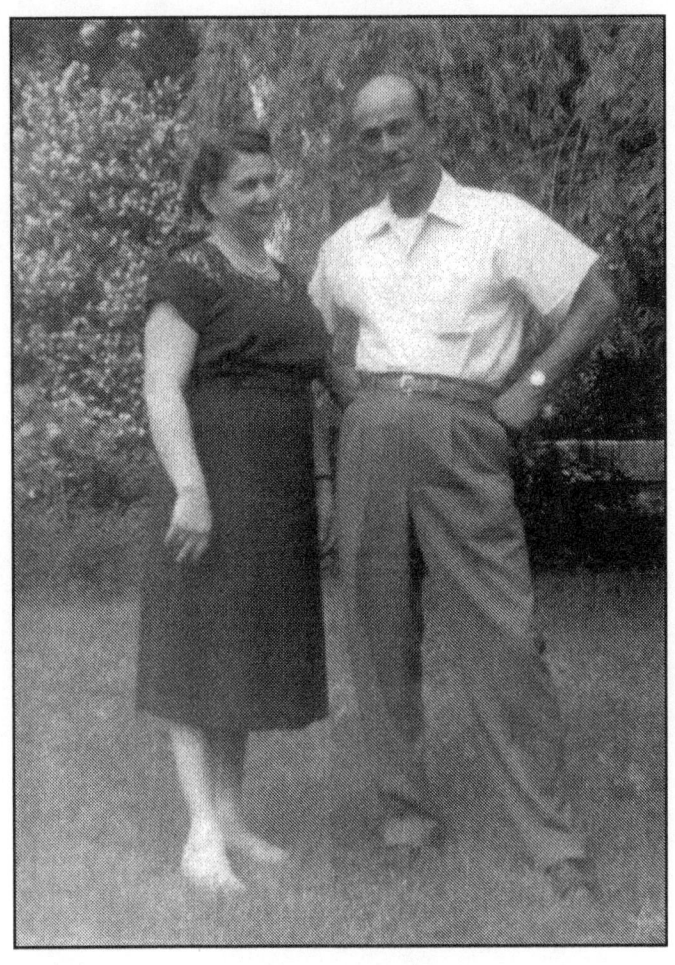

IN MEMORY OF MY PARENTS
GERARDO VERNA
AMELIA CAESARONE VERNA

thank you for showing me the true meaning of unconditional love.

Home

Direct the wind to me
Let it caress me
As a man with desire and Passion
I feel its strength as I become vulnerable

I let go and feel the peace and love I once knew
For that brief moment I meet my equal
And I remember the love of HOME

I woke up to the same hassle today as every other day in my life lately. Meetings, appointments, conference calls, and trying to set up a time to meet with my bozo manager.

I am fifty-four years old, divorced after twenty-seven years of a difficult marriage. I had never been given the opportunity to grow as a person or to be given a choice of a career. I seemed to have stuck to the same pattern I had always known in my life since I was a child. I have three lovely children that I managed to get out of this marriage. That in itself was all well worth it.

I had so much to accomplish and so many things to bring into my life. Life seemed to be passing me by and I was not getting it. Time was also running out and I was still working my ass off trying to make the money I thought I deserved in life. Focused on the trips I would be taking but somehow never did—the house in Tuscany I kept talking about, but I had no idea how I would get to Italy to see Tuscany; and the house in Rhode Island by the beach that I would get at a bargain and do the fix-up so that my family could have the get-togethers they never knew while growing up. Lord, I want to put twenty-seven years lost into my life in just a few years. What was I thinking?????

Got up, took my shower, got dressed, and off I went. I tended to put my bills aside, as that was the one thing I just couldn't make time for. Came home later that day, changed, and off to my spinning class I went. While I was sipping on what had become my daily glass or two of wine these days to relax at the end of my crazy days, I noticed an envelope from the breast center in the pile of bills on my dining room table. Curiously I opened it just to be sure my breasts were healthy before I tossed the results away in the trash. I had forgotten about the mammo I had taken and completely put it out of my thoughts or worries until I noticed the return address on the envelope lying on top of my pile of bills. Oh shit—I needed to go back for another mammo. Like I had time for this shit in my life these days. I had had return mammos for the last five years. Why did they even bother? I was perfectly okay. God forbid something was wrong. I called and made an appointment.

The appointment was the following week. The day of the appointment, a bad snowstorm moved over Connecticut and covered the state with a blanket of snow. I received a call from radiology and was asked to come in earlier that day. My appointment had been for 6 p.m. and I was already thinking about canceling as it was cutting into my spinning class that evening. The radiology group was on my way home and I was leaving due to the storm that moved over us. I took the earlier appointment to get this over with.

I couldn't quite put my finger on it, but I had a sense of unease this go around. I wasn't worried, but something just did not feel right today. Once the x-rays were taken of my left breast once again, I sat reading a magazine. The only choices of magazines seemed to be the "gossip Hollywood" kind. The room they had me wait in was so small you couldn't turn around. I was getting a bit nervous, as the storm had been getting really bad when I'd arrived and I had no idea how bad it was outside at this point. Not to mention I had heels on and had left my boots at home. Finally I got word to get dressed but not leave just yet, as the doctor wanted to speak to me. Great, just what I needed that day.

I walked into a dark room with the doctor sitting in front of my x-rays. Not a good sign. The doctor proceeded to explain to me that there were some calcifications he felt uncomfortable about, as there were one or two many of them. The doctor pointed them out to me and explained that my breasts were dense and he didn't want to worry me but that I would need to go in for a biopsy. He assured me it would probably be nothing at all, but let's take this precaution just to be sure. I agreed, and while walking out muttered, "So why do I need the biopsy if there is nothing to worry about?" I quickly dismissed any worry. My sister and a friend of mine both had had biopsies within the last year and they'd had nothing to worry about. Although unpleasant, they had turned out fine. The same would apply to me. Besides, I was in great physical shape and had no health problems other than an occasional relapse of Lyme disease. I could do this.

I didn't have to wait long for my biopsy to be done and for that day to arrive. Christina brought me to the hospital. I felt the biopsy was such a waste of time and the procedure was absolutely barbaric. I swear, a man had to come up with this procedure. No woman would torture another woman in this way. My biopsy procedure was taking place at 2 p.m. I could not eat or drink after 7 a.m. that morning. That meant no COFFEE. By the time I got to the hospital, I had the worst caffeine headache. I was prepared to take Valium until the nurse brought in an IV drip. I passed on the Valium once I saw it was not in pill form but rather an IV. I could do this without drugs. How bad could it be? Hospitals seem to complicate everything. I was brought into a room with very pleasant technicians. I was asked to lie down on a board with two holes for my breasts to fall into. I would have laughed if I wasn't so nervous about the whole procedure. Of course they had to explain in detail what was going to take place during the procedure prior to starting. As if that weren't bad enough, they remind you step by step what they are doing while you are going through the procedure. Like I couldn't feel it and figure it all out myself. I wanted to hear the words "We are all done and you are perfect. You can go home and never have to come back." I wasn't left with any doubt of what they did to me that day. I truly wish I'd had the option to pass on all the knowledge. This is a case where what you don't know won't hurt you.

I had wished they'd just knocked me out. I came close to passing out several times. I felt the needle go into me. Just knowing I had a needle in my breast and that it was going to suck out five areas was way too much knowledge for me to keep in my head while undergoing the biopsy. The caffeine headache was getting worse. Especially in the position I had to lie. My head was throbbing. I kept telling myself to hold on. I could run to Dunkin Donuts in the hospital as soon as this was all over. I needed my caffeine fix badly by now.

Finally the needle was taken out. The first try was successful and I was done. Once I got up to do my last mammo to be sure the staple was placed correctly just in case I needed surgery, I became very weak. What did they mean, another procedure? If I didn't need surgery, then did I walk around with a staple in my breast for the rest of my life? Did it come out, and when? Before finishing those thoughts, I passed out. I should have opted for the Valium.

Once they brought me back, the doctor sent a nurse to Dunkin Donuts for a coffee and muffin. The coffee was gone in minutes. I felt better after I ate the muffin. I was allowed on my feet, got dressed, and left with Chris for home. I tried to share my experience with Chris on the ride home but she wouldn't have any of it. It was too much for her and she was getting queasy.

I took two days off from work and I was back to my normal lifestyle again. I was once again putting all out of my mind as if I had nothing going on with me at all. None of this had really happened to me. I was just fine. I had wine once in a while, never smoked, tried pot a few times in my whole life, but that was the worse I ever did. I exercised and ate great. I stayed in shape and loved sports and any activity that challenged the body. I had become addicted to spinning. Nothing could possibly go wrong with me.

Trust In Your Spirit

Surgery is of mortal thought
Only when one cannot heal oneself should this process be
accepted
I have kept myself pure of thoughts and toxins
Drinking antioxidants—eating correctly
Staying within a peaceful grace
Allowing my higher power to deal with my earthly issues

I take from nature its nourishment with gratitude
The connection is allowed to deepen so that the medicinal process
can take place

Step over that line slightly to bring forth what is needed
My mortal self would not know

*Nature for nourishment

Trees
Birds
Animals
Ocean
Butterflies
Spiritual living
Surroundings kept pure by instinct

I received a call from my OBGYN. I had been working at home and Charles called me to let me know that the biopsy results found ductal insitu carcinoma. Charles is an absolute doll. I think all of his patients are in love with him. He's handsome in a California kind of way. He has a way about him that no other doctor has. Charles makes you feel as though you are the only patient he has and you matter; he cares about you and what happens to you. Charles makes all of his patients feel this way, but you seem to walk away thinking you're the only one. How could you not love and trust a doctor like Charles? He has shoulder-length blond (going grey) hair; wears sneakers; throw a little bad boy look in the mix but yet such a loving disposition and you end up with Charles. He called me that morning to explain what the diagnosis was for my breast results before the hospital could get a hold of me. He thought they might freak me out by telling me I had breast cancer and then giving me the explanation. I agreed with Charles that once I heard "breast cancer," I would freak and not hear them explain what stage I had and what it entailed moving forward. The fact that Charles used the term "pre-cancerous cells" kept me at ease through the whole process of the next few months. Charles suggested I see the same surgeon as his wife as she had gone through breast cancer years earlier. If Dr. Myers was good enough for Charles to send his wife to, then he would surely be good enough for me.

I called Dr. Myers and made an appointment. He took me within days. I liked Dr. Myers immediately. He had a sense of humor but was thorough, and there was an honesty about him. I felt relaxed with him. The first thing I asked was if I would lose my hair or teeth. How little I knew what was in store for me. He laughed and assured me I would not with radiation. We looked over his schedule, and he had an opening within a few days. He looked over at me, and I said, "Let's do it." This was great, as it didn't give me a chance to think it over. The only decision I had to make right then was whether I wanted a full or a partial mastectomy. That was no decision as far as I was concerned. I'll keep half the breast, thank you. Dr. Myers stated that the breast would not look bad at all once healed. Only half of me believed that one. I had been proud of my breasts all my life. My ex used to tell his friends that he'd married me for my breasts. I left the doctor's office and as I started my car a thought went through my head: I'll bet the ex is going to breathe a sigh of relief that he is no longer in my life. He wouldn't have to endure this ordeal and he wouldn't have to be stuck with a wife who would end up with a weird-looking breast. Why that thought would have even crossed my mind, I didn't know. I think the reality of what I was in for was starting to set in. The reality of what I was starting to think of myself was setting in.

The day of the surgery arrived. My daughter Erica took the day off from work to be with me. I felt as though she was the mother and I the child. She tends to have that effect on me quite often. Sometimes we do too good a job raising our children and they turn into us and they at times become the mother figure and we the child. I'd tried to escape the ordeal I was in for, but Erica would not let the denial set in. She needed me to understand how serious this was, and I didn't want to have any part of it. The whole time I was in the hospital, I felt as though I was not the one undergoing this surgery. It might have been the first real hint of the denial I would carry for the next few months. I remember at one point looking at Erica as I was lying with the IV in my arm, getting ready to go to radiology prior to the surgery, and I said, "I have no idea why I'm going through this. There is no cancer in me." I just didn't want to give in to this crap.

I was prepped for the surgery anyway and was wheeled into radiology for one of the worst experiences of my life. I had no idea what I was in for, nor could I have imagined I would need to have a needle stuck into my breast to the location of the staple that had been placed in my breast during the biopsy. At this point you have no options for painkillers at all as I'd had with my other procedures. There is a good reason for this, but my head shut off to the explanation once I was told what was about to happen to me with no drugs at all. I was a trouper, though. I could do this. The needle was placed into my breast by a doctor whose face I will never forget as long as I live. I would probably have nightmares of him after today. Once the needle was in place, I needed to sit there until the doctor read the pictures he had just taken, to see if the needle was in the correct position. My thought was, "What if it isn't? No way am I letting them try this again on me." I'm still holding on strong at this point. They needed to be sure the needle went far enough to the staple, as this would tell the surgeon where the area to operate would be. After what seemed to be an eternity, Dr. D returned to the room. I heard him say that they needed to get the needle in deeper. I think this is about when they lost me. Once the needle was positioned in the correct location, a wire needed to be inserted to point out the area that needed to be removed by the surgeon.

Once this procedure was done, I didn't care what else happened to me. I was getting twilight sleep now and I needed the drug badly at this point. Put me out and please don't tell me what else you are going to do to me today. I just don't want to know, I just can't know any more. Just do it and get it over with, please.

I was rolled into the operating room. Within minutes I was out. Exactly what I wanted at this point. Once the surgery was finished, I was brought back into the same room I'd been prepped in. I was awake at this point. I looked over at the chair next to me and saw my clothes I had worn when I'd arrived at the hospital that morning, before I'd had to change into the "hospital gear." Well, I was not about to wait for someone to tell me to get dressed. I wanted the hell out of here. I got dressed, they got Erica for me, and I was wheeled out of that godforsaken place.

Through the recovery of the biopsy and the surgery, I was in great spirits. God had chosen to have this cancer found at such an early stage that the process would be a piece of cake and I got to keep half of my breast. How bad could that be?

I became aware of something the day of my surgery. It was funny how Erica always seemed to need me and got so nervous when things went wrong or she got a bump in the road of life and today she just took right over for me. Erica was so protective of me. She wouldn't leave the hospital as I had asked her to while I would be in surgery. There is a huge shopping mall right across the street from the hospital. Now, you need to know that my daughter is a shopaholic. No way around it, so I thought this was great. She could get her mind off of me and go shopping for a few hours. Erica sat there waiting for me as a mother waits for her child when hurt.

I was proud to know that Erica had this inner strength when she needed to draw on it. I know that someday when Erica needs strength and I may not be around, she has her own inner strength and will use it to get through. She just chooses to lean on me while she has me and that's okay.

That evening I recall sitting on my couch looking back on the day I was ready to put an end to, and no one could wipe the smile I had on my face when I thought of how Erica had made her mom so proud.

Precious

God sends us love in the most precious parcels

"Bailey"

I felt so positive about my breast cancer experience that I didn't let it stop me from doing anything. It was as though I'd had a tooth pulled and I was back at work in no time. I attended a meeting in my office three days after my lumpectomy. I felt this was important for me, as I would win over a huge deal I had been working on. This could possibly pay for all my out-of-pocket expenses I managed to pile up during my last couple of months with breast cancer. I guess it didn't occur to me that I would be on short-term leave while undergoing radiation and this money I needed so badly would be in another rep's pocket in my absence. I still didn't get it, and I didn't want to let go. I talked the talk alright, but my head was still up my ass, so to speak. The only positive was that God was sparing me the worst, and I needed to take a good look at my life and make some changes fast.

I continued to work, thinking I would work through my radiation treatments as well. I wasn't keeping in mind that the company I was working for had just merged with another telecommunications company and NO ONE knew what the hell they were doing. I was in the Public Sector Sales with an idiot for a manager. I had no direction from management, and the issues that were taking place were costing me my commissions. I took a good look at the situation. I was working my butt off and not being paid for it. My manager didn't care, and *his* manager didn't care. I decided to go on short-term leave if for nothing else to get away from all the stress and bullshit in that company.

I was starting to feel alone with all of this now. I had a companion in my life, but something was missing. Rich had never been married and never made a real commitment to anyone. I would have to say myself included. I had been seeing him for over four years but there was always a distance between us. I couldn't remember the last time we had been intimate. This was worrisome to me, as I felt he may not know how to deal with intimacy and only one and a half breasts after this journey ended for me. He seemed disinterested in me with two great breasts. This would always be in the back of my mind. I assured myself he loved me, as he knew I had breast cancer and knew I was removing a good piece of my left breast, and still chose to stick around. I didn't dare tell him I needed more. I didn't dare tell him what I was going through inside. I kept a stiff upper lip for everyone—tried like hell to hang in there.

I buried the fear of dealing with radiation and what I may have ended up looking like after all of this was said and done. I knew the radiation would take its toll and I knew my breast was getting so beaten up that I didn't know what to expect once I was healed completely from this ordeal. At this point I felt as though I would never be healed. I wanted to be held and told I was beautiful. I wanted to be told it didn't matter what my breast looked like after this. I wanted to be told he couldn't live without me and he was thankful that all that happened was my losing a part of one breast. I wanted to be told that this blasted him open and he realized what losing me would mean to him and he thanked God I would still have a chance to be in his life. I wanted to be told by Rich that he wanted me to be a part of his life.

Nothing changed in our conversation. Rich was Rich. He had been alone all of his life with no real long-term significant relationship, and he was not about to step into one now. Lord, not now. When women would walk by and he looked while I stood there with him, I wanted to cry out, "Will you ever look at me like that?" I couldn't possibly expect him not to look or appreciate, but hell, he had been doing this for four years now. I was going through breast cancer. Could he respect my feelings and stop it while I was undergoing all of this? What is love to Rich, anyway? I wanted to hear that no one could compare to what he feels for me. I was lucky if I heard, "Have I told you I love you today?" Somehow these words and the way he would say them didn't cut it with me at all. Not these days.

He did take care of my garden, as he knew I had grown to love it. It was hard for me to tend to my garden these days. After ten minutes in the sun, I would get very weak and lightheaded and needed to get indoors. He did go on the twelve-hour drive to and back to pick up our new pup, Bailey. Bailey was supposed to be our pup. Once I had Bailey home, I didn't quite see Rich as much anymore. Bailey turned out to be a bit high strung. The pup seemed to need attention 24/7. Eventually I was told by our vet that Bailey had an attention disorder. I really needed this at the onset of my radiation. We picked Bailey up the weekend prior to the start of my radiation. I had to believe God knew what he was doing by bringing this cute but high-maintenance pup in my life just as I was going to start the most difficult piece of my breast cancer experience. Slowly, Rich let me know more and more that he could not deal with a pup like Bailey. Yep, it was Bailey and me now. He was all mine. I was a bit angry that Rich could give me the impression that we would have shared owning a dog. This was a true commitment that came with a lot of responsibilities, and I felt this was all unloaded on me. This was not the most appropriate time to dump this on me either. Unfortunately for Rich—Bailey and I grew closer and I drifted farther and farther from my relationship with Rich. What a shame, I thought, as this had been the first commitment I'd had from Rich. Somehow I wanted to believe he was capable of sharing something with me, and once again, I was on my own. I was afraid to waste my energy letting Rich know how I felt, as he'd never quite get this. The things we find out while undergoing cancer are amazing. It does not let us escape anything. It puts all in our face and will not be taken away unless we deal with it. It's your soul saying, "You need to heal. You need to love and be loved. You need to be worth everything in life. You deserve it. Love yourself enough to allow it and do not settle for less."

So—I have found my love for now. I have a little man in my life. His name is Bailey. He's an English yellow lab and he is beautiful. I thank God for Bailey in my life at this time.

Angels

Angels show up in life at the times you feel you can't go it alone
Your soul calls out to the universe and asks that an angel be sent

You don't realize how vulnerable you may be
Your soul is your core and keeps you protected

At my soul's request—My angel was called Merrill

The thought and the word "cancer" didn't really hit me yet. I must have been in some sort of denial. It all happened so fast I couldn't keep up with what was happening to me. I was outside of my body just watching. I was numb to feel anything at all.

I was visiting Dr. Raxlen weekly to get my vitamin C IV drips. This was to keep my immune system strong for the weeks ahead while I went through radiation treatments. Dr. Raxlen had treated me years ago for Lyme disease. I have a long history with Dr. Raxlen as my doctor. Dr. Raxlen does his treatments a bit more on the unconventional side of medicine. I trust Dr. Raxlen with my life. I believe he did save my life while I went through my bout with Lyme disease. I run to Dr. Raxlen whenever there is a medical crisis in my life. He has seen me through my worst times. I have no doubt I wouldn't be where I am without Dr. Raxlen in my life. His appearance reminds me of Hippocrates. He has a serous side of him, but when he smiles he reminds me of my dad. His smile would light up a room. There is a kind of twinkle in his eye when he speaks to you. He has a gray beard that gives him such a distinguished look. I feel blessed to have come across Dr. Raxlen and honored to have him as my doctor. In a nutshell—I love him to death.

Dr. Raxlen suggested I get a second opinion. He suggested a top-notch holistic cancer specialist in New York and was kind enough to make a personal call to get me an appointment asap.

My girlfriend Merrill called to see how I was, and when I mentioned my upcoming trip to New York to see the specialist, she insisted she take the ride with me. I felt it was such an imposition, but Merrill would have it no other way. She was going with me and that was it. Bless her soul. She had no idea. We were in the Holistic

Center for eight hours that day. She sat quietly and read a book she had purchased a few weeks ago at a book signing we had attended together. She watched me being taken from one room to another and not one complaint out of her. She must have wondered what the hell they were doing to me. Merrill became much more than a friend that day. She became family.

I think this was the day I realized I had cancer. It hit home. I started to realize I had a serious illness and I was passing it off as some flu-type alignment. My God—I really do have breast cancer. I received my second opinion. Three thousand dollars later I had some decisions to make for myself. What treatment was I going to do?—the holistic treatment, the conventional treatment, or would I put the two worlds together? I had to go with my gut on this one. No one was going to help me with this answer. This one was all up to me.

It was nice to have Merrill with me on the ride home. She and I have known each other over thirty years. We lived next door to one another while raising our children. We have a long history together. We spoke about our lives then and in the past, how much we had grown as individuals and as women since those days when our children were young and we were married to our exes.

I was able to discuss my day at the Holistic Center. I had gone all day long with no food and water. I had been through all sorts of testing. I had acupuncture for the first time in my life. I allowed it because I trusted this Center. The acupuncturist was no fly-by-night person, but someone who really knew what he was doing. With all I had gone through and the information that was thrown at me, I could not escape the fact that there was something serious going on in me. It needed to be respected and treated in a serious manner. Denial did not have a place in my life anymore. I had a grocery bag full of supplements I would begin to take. It was such a comforting feeling to have someone on the long ride home that cared enough and loved me enough to do this day with me.

We had a very nice dinner at an Italian bistro when we got back to town. We never stopped talking. We discussed her interest in producing cooking shows on our local TV network. Merrill is such an intelligent woman. I believe she will be successful in whatever she pursues. She has a wonderful husband to support and love her. This is her second marriage, and I envy her. Andy absolutely adores her. I have known Andy over thirty years as well. No one can utter a bad word about Andy. He has such a sense of peace and love about him.

I was exhausted by the time we got to the restaurant. I was so hungry, I couldn't eat, if that makes sense. I ordered suppa de pesca. Within minutes I had a huge plate placed in front of me full of pasta, seafood weaving in and out of the pasta, and a whole lobster to top the dish off. I was too tired to even play with it. I had some pasta and had the rest wrapped for me to take home. I dropped Merrill off, and as I watched her walk to her back door I couldn't help but wonder if I would ever know what it was like to wake up to someone in my life that I knew wanted to be there. Someone that would leave me with a sense of deep love . I think the cancer thing made me take a long look at my life. I had left my husband, as I'd had no doubt that he had stopped loving me and I didn't want to go through life with someone who didn't want me in his life. Could I be there again? Where was Rich through all of this? I didn't believe he really loved me. He may have loved my spirit, but I came with it. Had I put myself in the same situation this go-around as I had been in my marriage? I seemed to be doing the doctor/hospital visit thing with my friends and children. Rich did offer, but I never got the sense that he really wanted to be there for me. I felt it was just an "offer," and I thought it might have been a relief that I chose to let him off the hook.

Trust

We have all been given a gift from God
Some of us have a deep trust in it
Some of us tend to lose it along the way
Always searching for what was lost
Not quite knowing what it is or how to find it

I have been blessed to trust my gift
honor it
and most of the time listen to it

I believe it has saved me many times

The next appointment I had was with the oncologist at the Cancer Center. I came to the appointment positive and left worried. I didn't like anything about this doctor. His manner, his conversation with me, which I could distract and get him off the cancer topic easily, made me feel very uneasy. He didn't seem as though he stayed focused on his work. I had no trust in this doctor at all. He did not explain my condition in terms that I could fully understand or make a good decision on the basis of. He looked like he was right out of medical school and a spoiled brat. He had such a cocky attitude for someone that young. It didn't matter how good he may have been. We should all remember that there is room for growth in life, and to think we are already there, as this young doc came across, was so wrong in my eyes. The things we get from out first meeting with someone sets the tone for the relationship. It wouldn't matter to me if he was the best oncologist on staff—I was not going to be one of his patients.

He kept bringing up a trial that he was overseeing for a pharmaceutical company. He would have loved for me to say, "Yeah, I'll participate"—the trial being that there were two pills to take for five years once the radiation therapy was completed, both pills having serious side effects. If I opted for the trial, I would not know which pill I was taking for five years, hence would have no idea what I was doing to my body. Did he think I was some kind of moron? Why would I do a trial for a pill that I had no idea I was taking, for not one but five full years so they could track serious side effects? Was it not enough I would be doing radiation? Was there not going to be enough poison in my body after the radiation? I knew full well it would take me forever to recover just from that.

Lord knew I would never be the same after this ordeal, and this doc wanted me to put more poison in my body but this time not tell me anything about it. Where was the common sense here? What was I missing?

When I finally said, "Let me think about the trial," just to move past this conversation, he acted just like a child being handed his first lollipop. I couldn't get out of his office fast enough.

I called Dr. Myers, my surgeon who had sent me to this young doc, and asked him to get me another oncologist. I may have come off as a complete bitch, but it was my life, my body, and I would have to form a trusting relationship with an oncologist for at least five very important years.

When I received a call back from Dr. Myers, he asked me to wait for just a few days. It seemed that the docs had a Medical Breast Conference periodically, and the next conference was in just a few days from our phone conversation. My condition was going to be one of the topics shared with the medical staff attending that day. Dr. Myers would have many opinions from other physicians, and he thought it best to give me the feedback and have me make my decision once the conference took place. I agreed, knowing that no force on earth would make me go back to the oncologist I had visited.

I had an appointment with Dr. Raxlen that week to get my weekly vitamin C IV cocktail, as we now called it. Dr. Myers called while I was leaving the parking lot right after my IV drip. He gave me a little feedback from the conference, and I informed him that I still wanted another oncologist. He respected my decision and made the call for me.

My new oncologist left me a message later in the day and stated she would be glad to take me as a patient. My first thought, as I chuckled to myself, was that I assumed Dr. Myers and the young doc hadn't told her about me yet. I set up an appointment with her for the following week. I was glad to know it was a she and not a he, for some reason.

During my conversation with Dr. Myers, he asked if I would do a routine MRI of both breasts. Of course my guard went up. Dr. Myers explained to me that the physicians at the Breast Conference decided that I would be a good candidate for a breast MRI. Little did I know that they had found more cancerous cells in other parts of my left breast than what they had originally found. It was decided to do more tests after the conference. He also explained that I had very dense breasts, and they wanted to be sure nothing was missed. The MRI would show much more of what was going on in my breast than the x-rays. I had no problem with the open MRI, so I said, "Sure, why not, as long as it's an open machine." I have a problem staying still in an enclosed MRI machine, always have had. "Nope" was Dr. Myers' response. "We can't do an MRI for the breast in an open MRI machine." Is anything going to be easy for me through this? I had to think about it. I had gone through more than I could endure in a very short time. I was starting to lose it at this point.

I actually did when I received the call from the radiology group at Midstate Hospital. The poor woman on the other end of the phone was just calling to set up the appointment for me. In one month I had lost count of the doctor appointments I had gone to, the blood work I had taken, the biopsy, the surgery, and all the procedures I'd had to go through to get to today.

NO MORE. I DON'T WANT TO THINK ABOUT TREATMENTS, I DON'T WANT TO THINK ABOUT CANCER OR DO ONE MORE THING OR DECIDE ON ONE MORE THING. JUST LEAVE ME ALONE FOR A WHILE AND LET IT ALL CATCH UP TO ME. I couldn't think about this crap anymore. I needed some time to myself to let it really all sink in. I couldn't set the appointment that day, but I later did call back to apologize for being so rude and did set up an appointment.

Thoughts

There is a world I speak to
No words exist
If you listen you will not hear
If you speak it will not be heard

Our thoughts penetrate the veil
To understand and be understood

The day of my oncologist appointment came and I was anxious to meet my new doctor. I was relieved, as this was the satisfying experience it should have been. I had a female doctor as I'd requested from Dr. Myers. Not that I have a problem with male physicians. I just felt I would need a bond with this person, as we would be in contact often for at least the next five years. I must say, this was the first time I felt I needed a female physician. Up until then, I'd always preferred male doctors. I guess when you have such an intimate serious illness such as breast cancer you tend to think differently about who you would like to treat you. I felt I would be more comfortable in not only being treated by but communicating with a female doctor when being treated for breast cancer.

Dr. Scorsonali was very thorough. She made sure I understood all that had been done, why, and what the procedure would be going forward. I felt she knew her stuff. There was a toughness about her that I liked. So, after all was said and done, I was finally pleased with my oncologist. She was about my age, attractive, and seemed like a pretty smart cookie. I liked her. That was all that mattered. She also understood the importance of a good mammo screening and being sure we saw and found everything, as she had the same condition I did: fibrocystic breasts. It is very hard to pick up on things happening within a dense breast. I liked that she showed me images so that I could understand the difficulty and why certain procedures were needed.

So, I made my decision to go ahead with the MRI; and, yes, the closed MRI would have to be done. I had already made my appointment, but now I was sure I would show up for this procedure to be done as well. I got the importance of it—I was good with it.

As I was leaving the Cancer Center that day, I had to hold back my tears. I looked at my surroundings and I could not feel like a cancer victim. I didn't realize it yet, but I would see the same surroundings for many days still to come. I felt blessed as I looked around. I saw a young woman come into the center for chemo. She had a gorgeous face and such a bright spirit. She walked in with such a smile, as though none of this was affecting her at all. She was lovely. I turned my head and a couple stood near me. They were at the reception desk waiting for her next visit. Her loving husband was stroking her, and I felt each stroke of love he would give her. He stroked her arm and back the whole time they stood there. There was so much love, it just broke me. I had all I could do to contain my tears in the office. I couldn't wait to get into my car and let it all out.

Once in my car, I just broke down. Somehow my problem was not the issue. My cancer had been caught early and all I needed was radiation. I felt guilty that I would be a part of this group every day. I felt as though I should be going to another side of the hospital rather than be with the seriously ill patients. I wasn't sure if this was a remnant of denial that I was still carrying or I was scared that it could be me next go-around. I also felt a bit lonely and envious of the woman who had been so deeply loved by her husband at the reception desk. I felt guilty again. Was I not learning anything? Here I was envying a woman who was battling for her life when God had given me a gift of catching this early and had given me life to live. That was a "big dope" slap for me. I thanked God. Obviously he needed me to experience this, and I was going to trust God with all I had.

Within a few days after my oncologist appointment, I was back at the hospital for my MRI procedure. I hadn't gotten a wink of sleep all night, worrying about how I was going to be put in that closed machine. Again, no food or water, as I was going to get a Valium IV. Christina's boyfriend, Nick, brought me to the hospital, as I was not able to drive home after the Valium drip. Nick is such a sweetheart. He and my daughter have been dating each other for over ten years. He's become like a son to me. I'm not quite sure what the relationship is with Nick and Chris these days. It has been so on-again/off-again, I don't ask anymore. All I know is that I love Nick, and if he and Chris ever separated, I would be devastated. I could cry just thinking about it.

Nick had a huge test to study for, so, Nick being Nick, he made himself quite comfortable in the waiting room of the hospital. His sneakers off, books all over the floor. One might have thought this was his own personal space with his name on it. I truly believe Nick felt it was. He made himself so at home. He joked with the nurses and of course they just loved him. I think they may have thought he was my son, and I let them go right ahead. As far as I was concerned, he had become family.

I was walked to the dressing room in radiology once again. After changing into hospital clothing that was ten sizes too large for me, I was brought into the room with the MRI machine. To my surprise, it was a huge donut-shaped machine, and not the capsule I had remembered from years ago. I did have an IV drip, as it was part of the procedure, but I opted not to take the Valium with it. After all, this machine wasn't so bad. I could do this without drugs. I just didn't learn the first time around, did I?

I actually did quite well. The machine was well lit and I could see the opening if I lifted my head and looked forward. I was placed on the table with two holes for my breasts and placed into the MRI machine. I was told to stay perfectly still. All of this was so hard for me to do. I've never known how to stay perfectly still, and this seemed to be what they were asking of me every time I had a procedure done. As I lay in the MRI machine, I felt air blowing on my face. This did help me get through the time I had to spend in that position. There were times a strand of hair would be tickling my face or nose and, you guessed it—I had to stay perfectly still.

Once finally done, I put my street clothes on and met Nick, just as relaxed now as I had left him. I felt bad that I'd dragged him with me to drive, as I hadn't taken the Valium and I could have driven myself home. I told him I'd opted not to do the Valium and apologized that I had put him out that morning. He said I was crazy not to take the Valium, as he would have taken anything they would have offered him. It was nice spending some alone time with

Nick, even if it was just a drive to and from the hospital. I'm glad he did come along. I didn't feel that he minded either.

Another procedure down. I was told I would be doing this every six months moving forward. Again, my cancer had been caught early. No room for feeling imposed on. The MRI came out negative. Nothing was found since the surgery had been done. I was blessed once again.

Mind Choices

The body and the mind may get tired
The spirit is apart from both
Keeping the spirit strong keeps a healthy mind and body

Many times I have felt the frustration that no one would
appreciate me
I felt alone in my moral being
I felt alone in allowing my spirit to guide me

Was anyone going to come along in my life and understand the
importance?
Was I not to share this secret and piece of my soul with another
mortal?
Did I maintain my principles and dignity—and for what in this
life?

Through this journey with breast cancer I began to realize
This life of mine was lived for me
It was not to give or share this with anyone
There was no mortal that need understand me or this way of
living

I was going through the process of learning how well by living
this life the way I have would heal me, keep me loving myself, and
keep my faith
Without this spiritual bond I kept and developed, I would not
know and trust my higher power as I do

This experience is not for nothing. I have so much to gain if I
continue to trust and stay on this path.

I believe it was at this point in my journey, when I spoke to the radiology doctor, that I started to feel like a cancer patient. Whatever that may be. I was told the serious nature of what I had been through and would be going through. Dr. Kratzner was very thorough and made sure all my questions were answered. He wanted to be sure I understood what the next steps of the treatment would be. I wanted to hear that after all of this, I would never have to go through it again. I wanted a promise that this cancer that had visited me was gone and I would be able to put this out of my mind, as it would never pay another visit to me. Unfortunately doctors cannot do that. Not with cancer. This disease seems to have a mind of its own. Again—I hung on to my trust and love of God.

Dr. Kratzner was a very gentle man. I had a sense of ease with this visit. I believed the doctor was top notch, and I walked away with a sense of trusting him. I was introduced to the staff, as I would be seeing them every day for the next six weeks. They did give me weekends and holidays off. I'm not sure if that was for my benefit or theirs, but it didn't matter at the time. It was good to know I would get a break in between weeks. The staff was wonderful, always smiling and cheerful. I should think this would be a qualification for working in the Cancer Center. The only name I remembered was Dave. I'm not sure what his position in the Center was. Dave was the very first person who introduced himself to me. He took all of my personal and insurance information. I have to tell you that the reason I remembered Dave's name was because he was the first nice thing to happen to me through all of this crap. He was young, full of life, always had a smile on his face, and he was gorgeous. The staff must have hired Dave to make the patients' day. Dave was the first person to greet you every day for six weeks when you arrived at the Cancer Center for your radiation treatments.

My first radiation visit was complete. This was just a meet-and-greet and an informative introduction to what was in store for me in the weeks to come. I was set up to do a CAT scan to map out the area that would be treated with radiation. I sat with the nurse and went over my supplements that I'd received at the Holistic Center in New York. The doctor would allow me to take some that would help keep my immune system strong, but the others were not going to get his approval. They might have interfered with the radiation treatments, so they got a thumbs down. I would have to stop the vitamin C IV drips at Dr. Raxlen's as well. I could start up again a month after my radiation was completed, but not during.

After my visit at the Radiation Center, I gave serious thought as to what route I should go. Should I go the holistic route or take the radiation treatments?

The one statement that stuck in my head was made by one of the staff at the Holistic Center in New York. I was told that if I had one shred of doubt or fear that would stay with me if I did not go with the radiation treatments, then that stress alone should be enough to make me go with the treatments. I did finally decide to do the radiation and listen to Dr. Kratzner. I stopped the supplements he told me to and the vitamin C drips until a month after my treatments. This was a huge weight off of me. Trying to decide what was best turned into a full time job for me. It was starting to keep me up at nights as well. I felt I had seen and had spoken to all the players needed and felt confident with my final decision. I had no idea what the hell I was getting myself into.

I stopped at my oncologist's office before I left the Cancer Center. Her office was across the hall from the radiation department. I was asked to give more blood. Procedures, procedures. They wanted to be sure they had a blood specimen prior to my radiation therapy. Didn't they have a gallon sitting on the shelf that they had taken from me already? I asked that they do a hormone receptor test for me. Man, I was getting bold, and I started to realize I had way too much knowledge for my own good.

While standing at the receptionist's desk at the oncologist's, I recognized someone. I said, "Carol, what the hell are you doing here?"—as if I could be the only one from Wallingford who got breast cancer. I asked if she was waiting for someone. Hell, I was way too young to be doing this. I couldn't imagine anyone else my age going through this. Not someone I knew. I was shocked to hear that she'd had breast cancer twelve years ago and much worse than I had. I did the calculation in my head. In twelve years I would be sixty-six years old. I guess I could deal with it better if it were to come back at that age if I had to. Who the hell was I kidding?—I don't ever want this again; there will never be a better time. I WILL NOT EVER HAVE TO DO THIS AGAIN.

Several days later, I had a visit with Dr. Raxlen. It was to be my last vitamin C IV drip until after my treatments. Dr. Raxlen had a concern that my Lyme disease would kick up again, as the radiation would compromise my immune system. I'd had a horrible bout with Lyme disease about thirteen years prior. I ended up with a pick line in my arm for six miserable weeks. I was one of the lucky ones who needed it for only six weeks. I ended up with chronic Lyme disease. I have had some relapses, but no major crises. Man, I'm done with all of this crap. No more Lyme disease, no more cancer. I get it— God has a plan for me. I just need to figure out what it is.

As time was getting closer to start the radiation treatments, I was a bit edgy. Erica, being the typical college brat, was really getting under my skin. I'm sure she was going through her own silent concern over my health and trying to deal with college and keeping up with her work schedule as well. I wanted everyone around me to stay bubbly and upbeat so I didn't slide into a bad space. Erica was being Erica. It just was not good enough for me. I had a huge fight with her one evening and kicked her out of the house. She spent the night at her dad's. It was a well-needed rest for me. I needed to be alone that night. Didn't anyone get what I was going through and what I had to deal with? Didn't anyone know I was scared to death of the radiation treatments? Didn't anyone know I was afraid that my finances were starting to suffer from all my cancer bills? I would be taking a short-term leave, and not much income would be coming into our household. How was I going to pay for everything, including the out-of-pocket expenses I had accumulated while going through this ordeal? How could anyone dare give me a hard time now?

How could they? How would they know what I was going through? I acted as though nothing had changed in my life. I was going around telling everyone that the "bad breast" looks so good I may want to get the other one done. It was so swollen and looked so firm, with no visible scarring at the time, due to the swelling, that I was pretty okay with it. Hell, I could deal with this. I kind of liked the new size better. I was fooling everyone, including myself. I was getting a hint of how this was hitting me as each day passed. I needed to take a healthy look at how I was dealing with this. I felt blessed, but I needed to stop dismissing what was happening to me. I was right up against that edge now.

I managed to get through all the procedures without too much trauma, but the thought of going through radiation troubled me. What radiation was going to do to my body scared me. I knew the effects would linger. It wasn't like the surgery that would heal and I would be fine. Radiation was poison, and it just doesn't heal and leave in a few months. You're healing from this sucker for years after. I also had to visit the Cancer Center every day for six weeks. Cancer was all around me. I was given a sticker for my car so that I could park in the cancer patient parking. There was no getting around it, I was a CANCER PATIENT.

I was brought into a room for my CAT scan to be done. I was a ball of nerves at this point. No pain was involved with this procedure, but this bumped right up to my starting radiation. It was the final preparation to get me ready for my treatments to begin. Again, everyone was so pleasant. Martha, the CAT scan technician, was a perfectionist. This made me feel confident about her. Martha looked like she was in her forties. She seemed to be serious about her work and took pride in doing it right. I liked that she was a gardener, and she spoke of her family while bringing me through the series of preparations for my radiation. It made me look at her as a person and not just one of the staff.

The CAT scan took a while, as it was important to get the cast made and map out the area that would undergo radiation treatment.

The area would be my armpit, my left side across to the bottom of my chest up to my collarbone. Lord, did this really need to be done with such a wide area being treated? The cancer was in an area in my breast, not my whole chest. I was told that the breast area is large and they wanted to be sure the whole area was exposed to the radiation. I couldn't help but wonder why they didn't treat my good breast if they were taking such measures to treat such a large area. What would stop the cancer from attacking the right side anyway? I let that thought go and put it in God's hands. This was something I needed to go through, and I needed to be a good patient and stop getting frustrated with the why and why nots. It was what it was. The staff knew what they needed to do. I was thankful I didn't need the chemo, as did some of the patients I took notice of.

It's funny; I never wanted to be tattooed. I didn't have a choice today. Yes, I was tattooed in at least four different spots. Only I would notice them, but they were permanent and would be a reminder to me of my experience with breast cancer. This should keep me in check. Each time I noticed them, I would be grateful. I would never forget the remarkable people that were coming and going daily in the next six weeks while I visited the center for my treatments. These individuals were remarkable because not one person complained about one thing ever. They may have a look of fear or sadness, but not one person uttered a negative word in those six weeks. If every one of us had some sort of experience in life as these patients had, to endure this disease, to struggle to survive with the grace and gratitude that I witnessed, we would be a much better world. A peaceful world with a great acceptance for what is, and not try to change it.

I worked in a corporate environment and would not return to the company the same person I had been when I'd left just a few weeks ago. Would I ever fit in corporate America again? Who really cared, anyway? I was going with the flow and would end up wherever I was supposed to be.

I left the Cancer Center for the last time before my radiation treatments started. Next week was the real deal. The only excitement I had in my life right now was picking up my pup in Pennsylvania that coming Saturday. I wanted to be sure Bailey was home before

I started my treatments. He was ten weeks old, and I couldn't wait to hold him. All I had was a picture on the website to go by. In a few days he would be part of the family. I would come to find that my life would never be the same again after Bailey came home.

Healing

Our spirit knows what it needs to heal
There is a voice that guides us

No doctor or medicine can heal the way a pup can
Starting a day with a little face licking you to welcome you into
life each day

There is no greater medicine

Thank you spirit for allowing me to know Bailey would get me
through this crucial time
With his love, his adorable ways and even his puppy mischief

I could not help but love this pup more each day
There was no time to think about anything but spending time
with Bailey

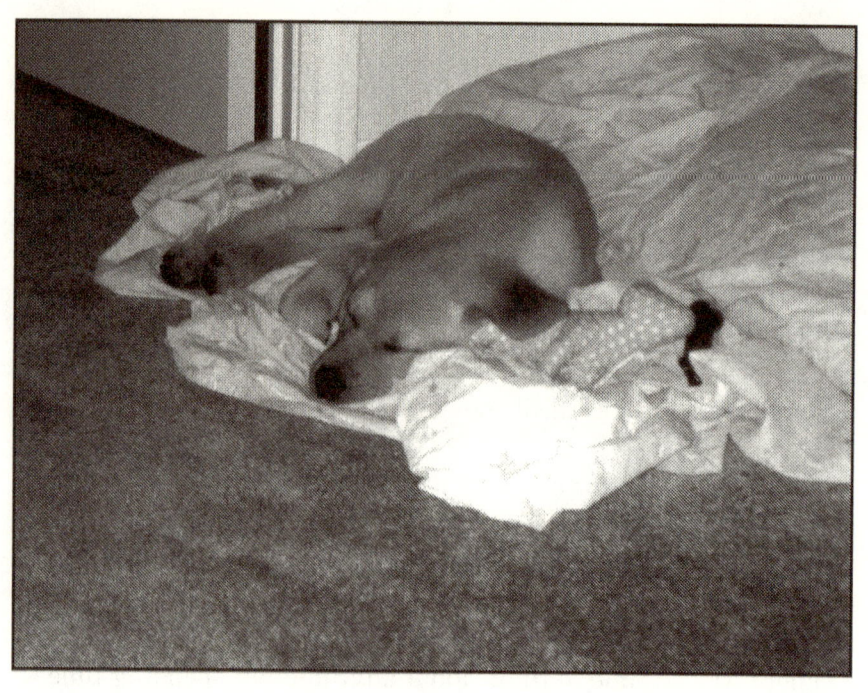

It had been weeks that I was searching for a pup. I was determined to find a yellow male English Lab. I called endless breeders, and not one of them had a litter, nor would they have one until the fall and into winter.

I did finally find one breeder that had a couple of litters. Rich, Christina, and Nick came along with me to pick one out. They were magnificent dogs. My favorites were Malcolm and Angus. Unfortunately all of the dogs this breeder had available were black. He would not have a litter of yellow pups that would be due to leave before July. Something told me I needed my pup now. I felt being on a short-term leave for a couple of months would give me some bonding time and of course training time. I walked away sad but still determined to find my yellow male.

I was not aware of how hard it was to find the exact dog you wanted when you wanted it. I called veterinarians in so many towns, I just gave up. All the breeders the vet gave me a list of had told me the same story over and over again. No litter for the next several months, and then I would have to wait eight weeks to bring the pup home. I did not want a pet shop pup; it had to be from a breeder. It didn't look like I had many options, and I was beginning to give up on the idea of owning a pup anytime soon.

I sat at my computer one night and endlessly looked for an English male yellow lab. I would find one and it would not be available, but they always seemed to have a black lab. I'd had to put down our family dog several years ago. Coco was a black lab— the most gentle dog you would ever find. He helped me raise my children. My youngest, Erica, will never get over the loss of Coco. I just wasn't ready to raise another black lab. I wasn't sure how the family would welcome another black lab and didn't feel it would be fair to the new pup.

Finally, there he was. The most adorable male yellow lab from a breeder in Pennsylvania. He was the pick of the litter, but the individual that wanted him had had a change of heart. He became available, and I just got a hint that he was the one. I called and left a message and sent an e-mail to follow up that I wanted him. Whatever the price was and however long the ride was, this pup was to be mine.

I hadn't heard from the breeder for almost a week. The breeder and her family were on vacation and were not able to get back to me sooner. The breeder informed me that there were many requests for the pup, but mine was the first request she had taken on her answering machine upon arriving home. She decided I would be the owner of her pup after a lengthy conversation on the phone, answering questions and filling out a questionnaire that she sent along to me via e-mail. It was Thursday and I was due to get the pup Saturday. I remember having driven to the beach with Rich that Thursday night, and all I kept feeling was I knew this was my dog. I could see the fire in his eyes, so I knew he would be a handful. The breeder told me the pup was very laid-back, but somehow I just knew better. It's all in the eyes. I couldn't get the pup off my mind.

Of course, my girls and Rich wanted to take part in picking out the name. "Bailey" seemed to be the only one we could all decide on, so Bailey it was. Erica wanted "Bruiser," and this seemed to end up being Bailey's nickname after we got to know him. Erica would later call him Pookachoo. I could see the embarrassment in Bailey's face when she called him Pookachoo at first. By and by he would become accustomed to being called Pookachoo. Even I would eventually slip and call him Pookachoo myself. Sorry Bailey, it just stuck.

Saturday came, and as I got up and looked outside, I saw it was pouring. The weather report stated it would rain all week. This was going to be a great ride to Pennsylvania. Not only was it going to take us over six hours to get to our destination, but we were going to do it in the pouring rain. I knew Rich wasn't thrilled about this venture, but he was good not to complain.

I drove up into Pennsylvania and I let Rich take over from there. We stopped at a diner for a late brunch. I felt like I had gone back in time. I was sitting in a diner back in the 50's. These people had never moved ahead. I had to admit that the food was great. I enjoyed the break from sitting in the car for such a long drive. We were still over an hour away from getting Bailey. It just seemed endless. As a matter of fact, the mountain we needed to drive over was called the Endless Mountain, and we were going to Endless Mountain Labs Breeders. Rich and I quickly realized why the mountain took on this name. It was beautiful country, but it was hard to enjoy it in the rain.

I was not feeling in the best of spirits that day. The fact that I had been through a lot of procedures and surgery and not slept very well the night before really wore me down. Finally we got to Endless Mountain Labs. We didn't get to go into the kennel to get Bailey. Rich and I waited in the house while the breeder went to grab him for us. Bailey was wrapped in a blanket like a baby, and when she handed him to me, he had this look of horror on his face. My first thought was, "Oh shit, this isn't the best reception I could have received from this pup." I quickly handed him over to Rich to play with and filled out and signed the paperwork needed. When I looked over my shoulder, Rich and Bailey were getting along just great. This put me at ease. It was very quick. It took no more than twenty minutes of our time to get everything taken care of. I bought his supplements that he would need to take and a huge bag of dog food so as not to change his diet, and off we went again for a long six-hour ride back home. It was still pouring out.

I picked up my pup and carried him off into the rain. Once I got into the car, I laid Bailey on my lap and there was an instant bond. I petted him and caressed him for the whole six-hour drive home. I fed him out of my hand, as the breeder had told us she had not fed him that day. She also told me not to feed him until I got home, but the poor thing was so hungry. Rich and I made many pit stops along the way to be sure Bailey was comfortable. His stubbornness was already showing. He would sit in the rain looking up at me and refuse to relieve himself as I stood there getting drenched. His little eyes looked up at me thinking, "You fool, why are we standing in this pouring rain?" The rain was relentless. It would have been an absolutely beautiful ride had it been a sunny day. The countryside was gorgeous. I would never see it again, as this was not a ride I planned on taking again anytime soon.

We finally got home, and I opened the front door to find I had my whole family waiting for me to welcome our new pup Bailey. I was not feeling well at all that evening. The ride had pushed me right over the edge. I could barely stand, I was so exhausted. I was glad to see that my family was such a part of this welcoming for me, but at the same time I wanted them all to leave so I could just rest and be with my new pup.

Bailey quickly became part of our family. I realized he would not just be my pup but would belong to the whole family. Once everyone left, I took Bailey and we went to bed. Yes, Bailey slept with me, and little did I know he would decide never to leave my side from that day on. Our bond just deepened as days went on. As I lay in bed that evening looking at him, I realized he had two markings on his back. Bailey was a yellow and white lab. He was primarily yellow on his back but he had two white markings, and when you looked at them, it looked as though he had wings. I liked to think this was a sign for me. He was my little angel.

He would soon be showing his horns as well. That night, we were both so exhausted that after everyone left, we fell fast asleep. Bailey bumped up right next to my legs. I thought it was the cutest thing. I wasn't alone anymore.

Beauty

Look within
Surface beauty disappears

There is a beauty of one's soul
Folded as a butterfly cocoon
Tucked away
Waiting to be allowed to come into its own

So deep in some it will take a tragedy
To step into place and become part of one's life

The tragedy being it was not allowed to flourish until now

———————————————

I started to see myself differently just before I started up my radiation treatments. My face was still mine but I couldn't quite connect to my body . Each time I showered, I would look at myself naked in the mirror and wonder where I went to. I use to like how I was put together, and through no fault of my own I felt a bit distorted. My left breast was now looking much different than when it was swollen. As the swelling went down, the scars and indentation became more visible. My left breast was now considerably smaller than my right breast. I didn't like it. This happened to me when I felt I was too young to deal with anything like this. Although I knew there were many women who had breast cancer younger, this was me. I still looked and felt young, and this was going to take some miles off of me quick.

If I didn't like it, how was anyone else going to accept me? This was truly God's way of making me look deep within myself. I am not all about breasts and a nice body. I am not all about getting noticed by men. I am so much more. I would never allow myself to realize this, but again, God was knocking on my door. He was getting my attention and he was going to teach me to love myself in a completely different way than I had been all of these years.

The next several weeks gave me the time to do all the things I had desired to do but had never made the time for. I would start to write my book, and who knows, I might just get my cookie business started up again and try to get it to take off. I have three signature cookies and I have been talking about this business since the kids were small. My children don't even want to hear it anymore. It has been all talk, and I have come up with so many excuses. Now I was given the gift of time. Let's see what I would do with it.

I'd have to teach myself to look at myself as a woman who went through many trials in her life and stood strong through all of them. One who has risen above each obstacle that came in her way, and without turning to drugs or alcohol but instead turning to God. God has never failed me.

I was very nervous about the first time Rich might see my breast. I wondered if I would ever allow that to happen. I knew I had a lot of work to do to trust the person I would share that moment with. It was not all about my appearance. I would need to trust that Rich was being honest when he said it didn't matter to him. He had no idea what had become of me. He was disinterested in sharing this moment with me these days, so I left it alone.

I was up most of the nights leading up to my radiation therapy. I wasn't quite sure what was so scary about this for me, except for the unknown. I was letting my mind go wild and wondering how long before my next visit with cancer. I was told that if this type of cancer does come back, it comes back very aggressively. The thought of this made me face mortality. This was a subject I never wanted to spend time thinking about. Although I'd had loved ones who'd passed on, I would just put it out of my head. Now, I found myself filling out a questionnaire I'd received in the mail from our local funeral home. I had always been appalled by this crap when it'd come in the mail, and now I was filling it out and sending it back requesting a packet with information. My thought was that if, God forbid, anything happened to me, I didn't want my children to have to deal with it. We all die. No one escapes from death. I wanted to be sure I was cremated and not buried. I wanted it done my way. It became extremely important to me all of a sudden.

There was no way I could have this conversation with any one of my children. They refused to listen to me. As time went on, I became less and less fearful of the word "death." Once you see yourself thinking of your own funeral, you seem to allow yourself to face death and try to deal with the fear that comes along with it. Staying connected to God helps. After all, was there really death? I would like to think we are just going back to our Father's home. It is life—just not as we know it here.

Awakening

The awe of such beauty
A butterfly cocoon sitting still

In astonishment I witness the brilliance of nature
The colors—the grace—the beauty

I allow this gift of nature to reach out to me
As it chooses to be lifted upon my skin

I hand it with love to be given back
It has taken my worries, my torments, my fears
And all I have held inside
To start me on my journey of healing my heart and my soul

I watch as it takes its first flutter to freedom
It rides the breeze as it frees the pain I have trusted it with
To filter into the healing of nature

I see it flutter into its own
And thank God to allow me this experience

Though short—it has given me my beautiful symbol for life.
I will honor and keep reminded of a no longer existence
Of an old cocoon within me needing to be shed

Weeks before my breast cancer ordeal took place, I had this incredible urge to visit Magic Wings in Massachusetts. They have a huge building with beautiful butterflies living in surroundings created just for them. It was wintertime, but I was able to step into summer just by walking into the building. I really felt I needed it. I wanted to be a part of this and feel these gifts of nature. I had gone to a flower show several weeks before, and Magic Wings had a booth. I purchased a butterfly cocoon that day. It would resurrect to be a beautiful spicebush swallowtail butterfly.

The women at the booth told me about the site they had in Massachusetts, and this introduced me to the start of a very special experience. I wanted to spend some time with the butterflies fluttering and dancing around me. I loved it when they chose to land on me. I got lost in Magic Wings. It was like a fairy tale come true. It is warm, and you have beauty surrounding you everywhere you look. I took notice of the individuals who were chosen by the butterflies. Almost all of the children were wanted by these gorgeous creatures of nature. The butterflies must have sensed the purity given by the children. I felt honored to have several butterflies land on me that day. They would sit on my finger, and it felt as though they were trying to tickle me. I had one butterfly land on my hand and it would not leave me. It was as if it was trying to tell me something, but I didn't understand. I watched this delicate living piece of art on my hand and thought, "You are so beautiful—don't waste all your time on me—there are so many that would like to share you. Hurry off to someone else that needs your healing beauty." Little did I know that day how much I had needed that butterfly on my hand. It must have known.

Quite a bit would happen to me in the next few weeks. Just a few weeks after my visit to Magic Wings was when I got the call letting me know I had breast cancer. I'd had my cocoon sitting out in the garage until April 1. I'd brought it into the house and put it in the bureau I had in my living room. Not a day had gone by that I hadn't checked on it. Through all my procedures and preparation for my upcoming radiation treatments, I never failed to check on my butterfly cocoon. Toward the end of April, I checked and found it had turned very dark. I thought for sure I had killed it somehow. What could I have done wrong? Was I supposed to keep it moist? Why did it turn black on me all of a sudden? I was now watching it several times a day to see if anything was happening to it or if I really did kill it This was not going to be a good sign just on the cusp of my radiation therapy. I finally got a sense that something was happening to this dry, black piece of stillness at the bottom of the container. How could any beauty come out of this?

One afternoon I went by the bureau and noticed something. I was in awe. There was this gorgeous spicebush swallowtail that had emerged from this piece of black I thought was as good as dead. It was as though it had to die to really come into its own. I felt this deep connection. Is that what was happening to me? Did I need to be faced with an illness that everyone associated with death to rise above it and come into my own? Was this the reason for the sense of urgency to go to Magic Wings? Was I supposed to see myself in this gorgeous butterfly? Was I supposed to discard my past pain as the butterfly had discarded this dry piece of brown and black at the bottom of the container it had stayed still in for months?

I let it stay in the container for twenty-four hours. I then passed it into a larger container that I had added a sponge with a water and sugar solution to the bottom so that it could suck on it. Once I saw that this butterfly was fluttering and its wings were ready to take it to where it needed to be, I was ready to set it free. I knew I would kill the poor thing if I kept it captive. This spirit had to be free. This was the same day I was to start my radiation treatments. I had to go in for my test run. The first treatment is set up as if it were the real thing, to be sure everything is lined up correctly and you are ready to go and understand what will be taking place.

The only thing missing is the radiation itself. I got a thumbs up and the next day I was at the starting gate. I would do thirty-six treatments. I would be there every day but weekends and holidays.

When I got home from my test run, I decided it was time to let my butterfly friend go free. Its wings were strong, and I chose a sunny, warm May day with a slight breeze it could ride on its first day of freedom into nature. I took it on my finger from the container and asked that it take all of my worries and pain I'd held on to for too long. I asked that it accept my forgiveness for people in my life that had hurt me deeply and that I had hurt. I handed it all over to this butterfly and asked that I be healed. That it take all I gave it and cast it away from me. That this will be the start of a cleansing for me. My journey of healing my mind, my body, and my soul.

In a ceremonial manner, I lifted the butterfly with my finger from the container and thanked God for all my blessings. I handed the butterfly back to nature where it belonged and watched it. As it fluttered away, it caught a breeze and rode it for a short time. I would like to think it let the breeze take all that I gave it to heal me. Once the breeze cleansed the butterfly of all I had handed over, it fluttered away into the wooded area behind my house.

The next day I started my radiation treatments. This was for real. I was scared to death. The machine scared me today more than yesterday. I wanted a sign that God was with me and it would all be okay. I was set up perfectly and the nurses left me in the huge room alone to start my first treatment. The huge machine would need to be in two different positions. One position was over my head, and the next was by my left side. I was so afraid; I had tears running down my face as I lay on the cold table prepped for the first shot of this silent poison. A poison I could not hear or see but whose power I knew the consequences of. I had to lie perfectly still with my arms overhead. I couldn't even wipe my tears away.

I noticed that some tiles in the ceiling had paintings on them. Some had the sky painted on them, some the ocean, leaves, smiling faces, and many more. As the machine finished penetrating its first rays into my chest while overhead, it started to move to my left side for the second dose. I was looking at the ceiling, and there it was right over my head. A calmness came over me and I felt God's presence. There was no doubt that God had given me my sign telling me he would be there with me every day I was left alone in that room. I would never feel alone again. The painting right over my head was a spicebush swallowtail butterfly. The exact same butterfly I'd set free.

I felt so blessed.

Voyage

In our life we have many voyages
Some we choose for ourselves
Some are chosen for us.

There is a greater voyage in our lifetime when chosen by a higher
power
I believe my voyage with breast cancer was my greatest voyage

This was a voyage with spirit
As days went by
I learned more and more how to be still
I learned more and more how to listen
I learned more and more how to observe

And learned more and more that no matter how alone I was or
felt
This voyage was of purpose

I was taught to be patient and trust
That what needed to happen for me to come into my own
Was taking place right before my eyes

 It need not be pleasant or joyous always
I needed to be taught so I would appreciate what was yet to come
into my life
With all its significance and to the fullest that is possible in this
lifetime

I had six weeks to go in my radiation treatments and I had no idea what to expect. I was trying hard not to let my imagination run wild on me.

Bailey had made himself at home and was into everything. There was no way I could possibly leave him alone in any one room of my house without coming back to destruction. The crate I had ordered for Bailey hadn't arrived yet. Christina would help by coming over to babysit Bailey. She seemed to have no problem watching Bailey for me if she was in between her appointments during the day, if the timing was when I needed to leave for the hospital. The times my treatments interfered with Christina's appointments, I would ask the hospital to change my scheduled appointment for that day. I would always make some stupid excuse why I couldn't make it on my scheduled time. I changed my radiation schedule three times. I think the staff might have been a bit irritated with me but never showed it. They were wonderful. I finally settled for the 3:15 p.m. slot. It was the last available of the day. I thought this one would have worked out best for me.

The crate finally arrived. Bailey wanted no part of it. He was now used to having the run of the house and was not about to give that up to be cooped up in a crate. He had gotten too spoiled and was given too much freedom. Unfortunately Christina could not give her life up to be there for Bailey every day, so Bailey got introduced to the crate whether he liked it or not. I would leave Bailey crying and would arrive home after my treatments with Bailey crying. I felt awful and rushed home to Bailey every day. At this point he became more than a dog to me. He was my friend, companion, baby, and I loved him to death. I would be so happy to see Christina or

Erica at home when I got back from treatments, as Bailey would not have be stuck in the crate for any great length of time.

My first week of radiation treatment was tough. I had envisioned my flesh giving off a burning smell. I had no idea I would not see, feel, or notice a thing that week. I hated being alone in the large room. I hated the machine over me. The only thing I focused on was my butterfly overhead and God's presence in the room with me. I felt his presence keeping me calm. I was always able to count on God in my life. He would never let me down. I knew as the days went by that I would come to realize what he needed from me—better yet, what he had been trying to do for me and I was not allowing him in. I chose to busy my life so much that God hadn't had a chance to be heard. Until now.

The first week consisted of only three treatments. It turned out to be not so grueling. The worst part was leaving Bailey; so how bad could it be? As I sat waiting for my turn in the waiting room on my fourth visit, I noticed a woman who had her appointment just prior to mine once I'd secured the 3:15 p.m. slot. You could tell she had a very hard time of it. I wasn't quite sure what sort of cancer she was being treated for. She had lost her hair, which meant she'd had chemotherapy. She was very frail looking and had no color left to her. I wanted to speak to her so badly. She kept to herself. A week went by and I noticed her sitting across from me waiting for her turn in the radiation room. I quickly got undressed, put on my hospital garment from the waist up, and sat on the chair right next to her. Me being who I am, I struck up a conversation with her. She was so very pleasant. I looked at her face and noticed how attractive she must have been. She told me she had red hair but that it was now growing back dark. Her breast cancer was much further along than mine was. She'd done the chemotherapy for eight weeks and now was at the tail end of her radiation treatment. She had lost her whole breast and, as anyone would feel at the end of an ordeal such as hers, did not want reconstruction or to think about another procedure. She looked as though she needed the rest. I could respect what she was feeling. There is something about a woman going through breast cancer treatment. One would think that this would tear a woman down to nothing, but I see that it does the opposite. It builds a woman to become a true woman. She spoke lovingly of her husband, so that let me know she was married and did not have to do this alone.

I seemed to envy everyone who had someone close in their lives while going through this. This was the time I really would have loved to have had a long-term relationship and grown old with someone. Only that bond would permit you to trust the love and commitment that would be needed from a loved one at a time like this in your life. I would go home and watch the tail end of *Oprah*. I had Oprah and Bailey waiting for me.

I think the most important time of the day for anyone going through this journey would have to be at nighttime when you're supposed to be lying in bed with your loved one, being held and being told how much you are loved; that they are grateful to have you still be a part of their lives. Evening seemed to be the worst time for me. I would look over at Bailey and be thankful to have him, but he could not love me the way a man could. I had no one to look over at and say "hold me" or "I need to feel loved" or "I'm afraid to be alone" or "I feel alone, help me." I found this to be the hardest to get past. I hated going to bed. I was exhausted but hated entering that bed. It was such a reminder of how alone I was in life.

Each day I would awake to Bailey on my pillow right next to my face. He would either be licking me or resting his head on my neck. At that point, all I'd felt the night before went away. I was being loved and the best way Bailey knew how to. I was realizing how much Bailey was going to mean to me as each day went by.

My ride to Midstate Medical Cancer Center was now routine for me—every day at 3:15 p.m., and it was getting to me, as I was not a routine person. This was another test for me. I was being taught to change my ways. God seemed to be introducing me to all the things I had no tolerance for in my life. I had to learn acceptance and how to allow things not to bother me, as there are greater things to focus on in our lives.

I was now on a first-name basis with all the staff. I still enjoyed seeing Dave's smile every day. I started to look forward to reading the quotes on the chalkboard every day and tried to see how it related to my life. I would see the same individuals there every day. We all had our set times. Some were very friendly, and some wouldn't even look at you. I couldn't get their attention to say hi to them. One man in particular. He was brought in a wheelchair. He never spoke a word to anyone. I noticed him outside waiting for his ride one day as I was leaving after my treatment. He had just received his radiation treatment. I was told that he'd had chemo prior to his radiation therapy. There he was sitting in his wheelchair with a cigarette in one hand and a cup of coffee in the other. I wanted to turn around, walk over to him, grab the cigarette out of his hand, and say, "Why do you bother coming here every day? Do you care at all?" I just drove by him as I left the parking lot shaking my head. He had lost his will. It was so clear to me. I guess not everyone can change the way they live or their habits because one day they discover they have cancer. I was lucky I took this as a wake-up call. I wanted to see my children marry. I wanted to share in their joy. I wanted to spoil my grandchildren someday. I felt sorry for the gentleman that I had just driven by waiting for his ride and not really caring to be a part of any of this.

Each day became different but the same. Monday and Wednesdays I would get to visit with the nurse. She would check me and see how I was coming along. I got to know her quite well. We traded stories about our dogs. She shared the excitement of her new grandchild. She told me how her son was in Iraq. God knows when to send nice parcels in life. She received her grandchild right after her son left for Iraq. I tried to bake goodies for the staff when I was up to it. I wanted to show my appreciation to all of them. I felt they deserved to be thanked in any small way possible. I can't imagine how hard it is to come in on a bad day, as we all have bad days, and yet they still put on the happy face for all of the cancer patients.

I became exhausted by the first several weeks of treatments. I became lightheaded and nauseous. I walked into the treatments already drained. I had kept working and keeping up with everything in my life as if nothing was happening to me. I never really rested after any of the procedures or the surgery. I was taking the supplements but I didn't allow myself to rest. I simply do not know how to rest. Never have. Things were about to change. There were going to be a lot of lessons learned through all of this.

Mothers

There is a time in your life when you understand how important
your teachings are
A time when you look at your children and your heart smiles

You know they get it
Everything you have taught them
The things they would laugh and make fun of included

There comes a time you know and see beyond
Your soul knows that these children you have raised are exactly
what you intended to raise

My children get it
My greatest gift this Mother's Day was that I can be so very
proud of my work raising them, as it complements the individuals
they have become today

What greater gift for a mother than the gift of "pride"?

Mother's Day was the weekend that ended my third week of radiation treatment. For some reason my energy was starting to kick in. God only knew where it was coming from.

My son and his girlfriend Tenesha had moved back to Connecticut a few days after my lumpectomy. They didn't plan it that way, but it fell in place beautifully for me.

Tony had met Tenesha in New York City a year ago at a party with mutual friends. They had both hit it off. I knew my son was hooked when he called me the next day after meeting Tenesha and said, "Mom, I just met the most incredible person." It happened very quickly after their meeting, as Tenesha had just bought a house in Salt Lake City, Utah, to be with her family. She was moving from California where she had been living. Tony and Tenesha tried to carry on a long-distance relationship, and I could see Tony was not lasting. He needed to be with her. They had met in April and in July he was packed and on his way to live in Salt Lake City. Less than one year later, they had both decided to move back to the east coast. It was a compromise on both sides. I thought it was wonderful of Tenesha to be so understanding to move back to Connecticut to see how New England living would be. I couldn't have been more thrilled.

Tony and Tenesha wanted to have the family over for Mother's Day. I felt this was way too much for them to do. The expense and the work. You know how we Italian mothers think. It should be at our house or nowhere. I declined, as I felt I wanted to visit the Buddhist temple in upstate New York on Mother's Day morning. I felt it would be too much to do dinner afterward. Not only that, but

I might not be up to it and I would be leaving Bailey home alone all day long. We know how hard that would be on me!

Tenesha was determined to cook me dinner. She seemed to have the same stubborn streak in her as I have. She was so sweet about it that I finally caved in. We decided Tony and she would be over my house and do a lunch for me when I got back from the temple. I was very touched. It was a compromise. That Italian in me still needed it at my house.

Tenesha had decided to visit her family in Utah and was on the way to the airport, so it worked out beautifully. Tenesha had found a wonderful position in a publishing company in Old Saybrook and had a week before she started working. She thought this would be a great time to visit her family, as her sister had just had triplets.

Once Tony and Tenesha left, Chris and Nick stopped by. Erica had taken the day off, so I was able to spend time with all of my children on Mother's Day. Of course, Bailey was there to torment us. I couldn't have asked for a more perfect gift from my family.

It was the end of a very meaningful day for me. Rich and I drove up to the temple in upstate New York that morning. The temple was having a healing mass for Mother's Day. I allowed myself to do some visual healing with the chanting that was taking place in the temple. With each chant, I would visualize my cancer cells being beaten up, pounded and broken up inside of me. When the chant ended, a drum would sound. With this drum, I visualized the particles that had been broken down leaving me like dust would leave a dirty rug. Then came the ceremony of cleansing. We would wait our turn to go to the altar and pour water over a bronze Buddha. At this point, I visualized the final cleansing. I became the Buddha and poured the holy water over myself and completed my cleansing and healing.

It was powerful. So much healing and not one person had any idea what was taking place within me. God and I took care of me that day. It did not matter where I worshiped or the mass I attended. I was raised Roman Catholic but was no longer satisfied with the Catholic Church. I raised my children Catholic for my family's sake. They know I will support them however they worship. I feel I have given them the spiritual foundation. They need to find what feels right spiritually for themselves. As long as they carry God inside of them, they will stay connected. I believe we are all connected to one higher power. I felt I had a direct connection to God. God lives inside all of us. We are all his children. Breast cancer made me reconnect deeper than I had ever been. I walked away thinking to myself that I didn't need radiation therapy after my healing experience at the temple this morning. The mortal side of me said, "Stop being foolish and do all that needs to be done." I was healed on a spiritual level and now I needed to complete my physical healing.

Time

Six weeks can turn into an eternity

If only I could have been chosen to spend my six weeks in a villa
in Tuscany
How wonderful would that be?

I was chosen to spend six weeks visiting a Cancer Center
I don't ask why these days
I go with what I am suppose to do

Each day I awake I listen to the message given me
I cannot seem to escape a thing these days

All that may be wrong in my life is in my face
Each way I turn my face it seems to plant itself in front of me

My soul will be walking out of this ordeal with a clean slate
No drama, no issues, no hurt moving forward

To get there I would deal with pain. Ultimately the burden I
carried would be lifted
There will be no more doubts in my life. There is no energy that
need be wasted on doubt

Time was my gift
I chose to make every second count from this day forward

It wasn't until the end of the third week of my radiation treatments that I began to feel better. My energy seemed to be coming back. My spirit was up. I was not tired at the end of the day as I had become when I'd started my treatments weeks ago. I couldn't understand what was happening to me, but I loved it. Something told me I shouldn't be feeling quite this well with what I was going through these days.

I sat at my dining room table one morning of my fourth week of treatment. I took out the folder that held all my cancer information I had accumulated in the last several months. I wanted to read up on my supplements. Oh my God, here it is. Ambrotose. As I read up on this supplement, I was experiencing the effects of the supplement I had started to take when starting my radiation treatments. I decided that day that this supplement would be a must for the rest of my life. Lord, if I could feel this way while going through treatment, can you imagine what I'll feel like once this ordeal is over and I go back to a normal life?

I realized this supplement was something I believed in and decided I would sell it. I took that thought and tracked down the sales director, ordered my kit, and was excited about putting this information out there. It seems Connecticut had not been introduced to these products. What better way to make a living than to sell something you truly believe in, that you have a testimonial about and would help others going through their own health crises? Was this the answer to my getting out of a corporate world I had no business being in anyway?

I felt good enough to start getting out of the house and enjoying my friends. I made a call to Carol, the woman I had met at the oncologist's office who had shared that she had been cancer free for twelve years. I had promised I would call to get together. We made plans and had dinner at a restaurant in town the following week. We had some time to chat alone and her best friend joined us halfway into our dinner. Carol shared with me how wonderful her husband had been during her breast cancer ordeal. I could tell it strengthened the bond and love they had. She beamed when she spoke of how concerned her husband had been. Once again I became envious. I had no one in my life that was that concerned for me. Yes, my children were, but there was no man to support me with all of this. I understood how the loneliness was getting to me. I wanted to be loved and held. I wanted a bond with someone I knew would want and desire me no matter what I looked like after I healed from this journey. That what I looked like wouldn't matter. I could see that Rich would not come over much these days. I could see he wasn't going to be able to share this experience with me.

I had my children. Christina and Nick were over just about every day. Some days they would swing by twice a day. I looked forward to the visit, as they would help me with Bailey, who had more energy than I could handle these days. They would bring Christina's dog Nala and run the two dogs so Bailey would get tired out. Bailey hardly slept as a pup. I was starting to think Bailey had a disorder, as I had never seen a pup with this much energy or a pup that needed as much attention as Bailey needed. I was at my wit's end with this pup. I walked him several times a day and paid constant attention to him. I had to give him the attention or he would be into something as soon as my attention turned away from him. I didn't want to complain to anyone. I quickly saw that Bailey's behavior had a not so great effect on Rich. What Rich couldn't see was that Bailey's unconditional love was seeing me through all of this.

I hadn't really noticed much change in my breast during the first four weeks of radiation treatments. Memorial Day weekend was the start of my fifth week. I noticed my breast was quite swollen now. I noticed that the area of my scar was becoming a deep brown and that I had some brown specks all over my breast. I lifted my breast and it was really brown. By the end of the fifth week, I was itching so bad I felt like a dog with fleas. When I'd had no pain or itching, I had been able to put the breast cancer out of my mind. I'd needed to think about it only when I visited the hospital. Now there was a constant reminder. The discomfort was setting in and I still had two weeks to go. I was nervous now. What the hell was I going to look like once I completed all my treatments?

Rich surprised me that weekend by telling me he would build me a pen for Bailey in my basement. I thought it might be to get rid of Bailey when he visited, but it didn't matter. I needed somewhere to put Bailey other than his crate, as that situation was not working for me at all. It took Rich only one day to build the ten-by-ten-foot pen in the basement. Rich was exhausted by the time he was done and left as soon as he finished.

The next day Rich went kayaking that afternoon. I had the kids over for dinner. It was the evening before Memorial Day. It was a beautiful summer night and we ate outside. Rich stopped in for dinner but left immediately after. That night as I lay in bed, I allowed it to set in. Rich did not love me. I had been with Rich for five years and I felt like such a fool. I had been brave enough to show Rich my breast that morning before he had started on Bailey's pen. I'm not sure what I expected from him, but I felt as though I had shown a stranger my breast. I got an "it's not that bad" reaction, and that was it. I was feeling abandoned by Rich. He was cutting his visits shorter and shorter these days. There were no quality times, and I need them desperately now. More than ever.

Everyone had plans the next day, Rich included. He was off to his friend Chris's house for the day. I couldn't be in the sun and didn't want to put a crimp in anyone's day, so I stayed home with Bailey. Rich assured me he would be home in time for a picnic at the beach later that day, as he didn't want to have me spend Memorial Day completely alone. I was looking forward to this all day.

It was a gorgeous Memorial Day when I got up. I went about my usual routine. First thing was taking Bailey out to do his "duty." As I walked down the grassy hill on the side of my house, I got a hit of the sun. I could feel the warmth penetrating through my clothing. I had such a yearning to be like everyone else that day. I wanted to be part of a gathering and be able to sit out in the sun with family and/or friends. I felt so abandoned. Somehow an emotional state took over me. I could cry at the drop of a hat.

Rich was going to spend the day with his friends enjoying the water and the sun. He didn't even call me that morning before he left to meet his friends to see how I was. I spent the day with Bailey and being bored out of my mind. I tried to read or write, but somehow the emotional state I was in would not allow me to be able to focus on anything. I just wanted to be a part of something that day. The fact that my mom had passed on during a Memorial Day weekend added to my emotions.

Rich had said I would hear from him around 3 p.m. or so, and he would be back in time for a supper picnic by the beach. I hung on to that to get me through. It seemed an eternity, but 4 p.m. rolled around and I hadn't heard from Rich. I looked at the clock and it was 5 p.m. I still hadn't heard from Rich. Finally at almost 5:45 p.m., I realized I had been forgotten by him. Trying to hold back tears, I took Bailey and we headed for the beach alone. It seemed as though everyone was doing what they enjoyed doing with people they enjoyed being with and I was not going to be a thought in Rich's mind today. He called me while on the way to the beach and he just didn't get it. How could he? My life was the only life that seemed to stop dead for several months. I realized that day how alone I was. I reflected on my life and realized I was really alone. I had been alone in my marriage and now I was alone in my relationship with Rich. Had I done that good a job at being strong in life that no one realized I was human and needed love and someone to be there for me—especially now?

I had spent the previous evening with my children, so I did not expect them to stop by, although Chris and Nick did for a short while. I sensed they wondered why I was not with Rich, but they were nice enough to leave it alone when they asked.

Bailey and I hit the beach around 6:30 p.m. When I pulled into the parking lot at the beach, I could see I was not going to be alone at all. As Bailey and I walked the beach, I realized everyone was either with a huge group of friends and or family or partnered with someone. I was the only one walking alone with my dog. I wondered what I would have thought of me if I were in their shoes. I would have felt as sorry for me as I was feeling for myself. I didn't stay long, as I was fighting back tears. I couldn't get home fast enough.

After a phone conversation that turned into a fight with Rich several hours later, I ended the day, you guessed it—alone.

Rich seemed to stay away the whole next day and evening as well. I realized then how little he could deal with this, and I started to truly question what he felt about me. I think all the anger and hurt I'd held inside for the last few months came pouring out of me. When I finally spoke to Rich that evening, I got so upset that I took it out on my phone and with one slam broke it. I felt as though my skin was going to crawl off of me. I had no one to turn to; no one to hold me and tell me this was normal and I would be fine. The fear rose up within me and I had no idea what to do with it. In my heart, I felt that Rich should have been there. He should have put his feelings aside and understood that I was not going through a normal time this year, that every day meant something to me, and holidays were going to be very important. I couldn't believe he could have sat with his friends and not even bothered to call me to say he would be late at this time in my life. Not after he had made definite plans with me.

This was the start of the end of my relationship with Rich. I knew I could not expect him to feel or do what was not natural for him. I knew after almost five years that he could not and would never commit to me. He would promise me he would seek help and tell me he wanted to commit more than anything, but actions were stronger than words at this stage of our game. I'm sure he'd said this to many before me as well. Every day I would expect less and less from Rich. He was not able to be intimate with me and could give me no good reason. The red flag grew larger and larger. I knew this was not the time to make huge decisions, as I wanted to be sure it was my head and heart talking to me and not an unstable emotional state due to my ordeal of the past several months. Time would tell and soon enough.

Changes

One expects change in life
Never knowing what changes will resurrect

Our hopes are that changes are for the better
Some would look at my change in life and feel sorry for me

I take my change as a dramatic cry from my soul
Once you override that cry from your soul it resurrects in many
ways

Mine was breast cancer
My decision was to listen and not make the ordeal any more
grueling than what it would be

Keeping positive and walking in the grace of light
I have brought many new gifts into my life

I look at the gifts from my old life I would like to carry over
And cherish these gifts as gold

I would have to admit that breast cancer was my introduction
To a full and more peaceful life.

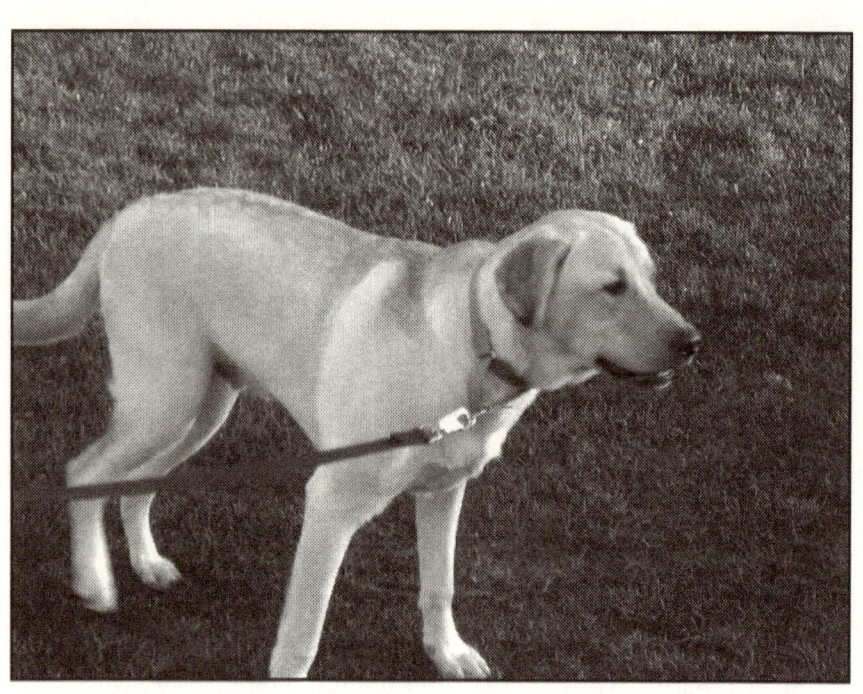

It was now the fifth week of radiation and I was starting to go downhill fast. Both Christina and Erica were sick with a bug, and I wasn't sure if I had caught it as well or this was what I was supposed to be feeling as my treatments progressed. Erica lived with me, so I was sure I must have caught whatever she had.

This was probably the toughest week I had to go through. I could see my energy wasn't quite what I would like it to be. Yes, it was better than what I was seeing around me in the Cancer Center every day, but I was not me at all. The effects of the radiation treatments were becoming more visible now. My chest area was so itchy, I couldn't sleep well. The undersides of my left breast and my left arm were sore and a very deep brown. I noticed that the skin under my left breast was starting to separate. The sweat from walking Bailey on our daily walks was irritating these areas. I had six treatments left. These were going to be the most difficult to get through. I had about had it with all of this by now. The trips to the hospital, the treatments at the same time every day, speaking to the nurses and doctors—I was cooked in more ways than one.

I had to find some humor in my experiences. Like the Saturday I got up and decided to go to the produce market down the street. They had the best breads and the freshest fruits on weekends. This particular Saturday morning was unseasonably cold. It was the beginning of June but felt like late October. Everyone in the produce market had heavy sweatshirts and jackets on. It started to rain before I left the house, and I should have thrown on a sweatshirt, but I was experiencing hot flashes since I started my treatments. I'm not sure if this was brought on by my menopause or if this was one of the side effects of the radiation treatments. I was so hot, the sweat kept pouring off of me. I threw on shorts and a tank top. I knew everyone would look at me and wonder what the hell was wrong with me, but I was hot with no clothes on. With no jacket or sweatshirt, I was on my way. Of course everyone stared at me in the market. At this stage of the game, I could care less what they were thinking of me. I wanted my specialty breads and the fried chicken cutlets they had in the deli behind the produce. I got a hint of how strange this breast cancer ordeal was making my life. I felt as though I had landed from another planet, and what worked for everyone else just didn't seem to work for me. I checked out my groceries, piled them in the back seat of my car, and drove off—windows down. I thought of myself walking through the market dressed in shorts and a tank top and chuckled to myself. What a freak I had become. This would only teach me to be humble. I could never question anyone after this experience.

I felt bad that I was not able to work on my garden as I had in the past years. I could stay out in the sun for only about ten minutes, and I would have to come in because I would get lightheaded. I had made a section of my garden in the front of my house my Cancer Garden.

Every Tuesday, Bristol Myers would send Midstate Hospital Radiation Department potted plants for the cancer patients. They weren't necessarily plants I would have gone out and gotten myself, but these plants had a lot of meaning. I would bring home four or five pots of flowers each week. They would be a reminder to me of what I was going through, the knowledge I had gained through all of this, and the changes that would have to be made in my life after this experience. I would never be the same person after being touched by cancer. I put them in a spot I would look at every day, as I wanted to remind myself of the better person I would become. My cancer plants were accepted beautifully by the plants that had already made a home in my garden from previous years—the plants that would greet me every spring and summer. I wasn't sure what I would do in this space once these flowers died at the end of the summer. Should I get a bush? I needed to have something with meaning in this space from now on. The next year I would sprinkle seeds consisting of wildflowers that would attract butterflies and hummingbirds. I wanted to watch the miracle of these small seeds forming plants that would move the dirt above it to grow into an area of beautiful flowers. They would be magnificent, and that next year they were flowers that I chose. I would come to find that this was exactly what I did that next year. They invited so many butterflies. This will always be a special section of my garden. It will always be a reminder to me of my second chance at life as it should be lived. A life that will make me happy and perhaps give back to the world a little bit of love and gratitude. If my positive energy would help others in my life, that would be well worth what I had gone through with my breast cancer. Bailey seemed to love running and jumping after the butterflies.

Bailey seemed to be growing so fast. He was now four months old and so clumsy. He would drive me nuts. He had so much energy and it was hard to keep up with him. I was at the end of my treatments and he had no idea nor did he care what I was feeling. He was a puppy, he wanted to go for walks and runs and have play time and he would drive me nuts until I gave in. I must say, he did keep me active these days. I was not allowed to sit around and feel bad for myself. Bailey pushed me into walking, running, and keeping active. I was not allowed to give in to breast cancer. At this point I decided Bailey needed to be put in his pen for longer intervals. It would not be long before I started back at work and he needed to learn how to be alone in his space. Besides, I needed my down time, and there was no such thing as down time with Bailey around. Our walks were not as brisk as they used to be now, and the running stopped. Everyone in the neighborhood knew Bailey, as we were outside most of the day walking. Everyone seemed to take part in watching him grow, and somehow I noticed there were more and more Labrador pups that were making a home in the neighborhood. Had my neighbors gone nuts? They should have asked me what I was going through with this pup. They saw the cute pup and owner sharing walks and how wonderful that must be to have a bond as Bailey and I had. What they didn't know was how crazy he was making me. Erica, Christina, and Nick had loved to spend time with Bailey until now. He was getting to be a handful for anyone, and he wasn't enjoyable to be around. This unfortunately made me his whole focus.

Bailey was getting used to his pen. I thought it would be a lot harder, but I think he might have needed his own space away from me as much as I needed my space away from him. Erica had picked up a book for me to read. She felt it would make me feel better with my situation with Bailey and relate to the author's experience with his dog Marley. The book was called *Marley*. It seems Marley was one of those "exceptional" dogs, as Bailey was. The owner narrated the lifetime of a dog that was a bit more "special," shall we say, than most dogs. As I read the pages, I related completed to this author. Marley was intelligent but had many issues that would test his owner. I seemed to have Marley reincarnated. I think Marley and Bailey were just so intelligent that they became bored very easily and needed to be entertained constantly or there were consequences. I would find that Bailey, like Marley, would end up being the best dog I ever owned. They seem to have a spirit that understood completely. A loyalty and love far more than anyone could ever ask for. They were both keepers, but we as owners were tested. I found that I was capable of the same love that Bailey was. The true meaning of UNCONDITIONAL was now a part of my life.

Bailey is my cancer dog. Bailey will always have a place in my life. I can't imagine what life still holds for me. Bailey was brought into my life at a time of many changes. To introduce this puppy into my life at this time was meant to be. It was one of the first things I listened to and acted on in my new life of changes. I can only thank God for the plan he has for Bailey and me.

The Test

Life will sometimes send challenges we think we cannot conquer
This is when we become one with mind and spirit to overcome all
obstacles

My sixth week of radiation was one of these tests
I was positive and stayed in tune with my spirit until the last week
I felt my body turning its back on my mind and spirit
My body cried out for help and I stood watching unable to do a
thing to help it

How could I explain that for one more week my mind, body, and
spirit would not be one
This bothered me more than anything I had gone through with
this journey

I always listened to be sure I was mind, body, and spirit as one

Now I could not be

I had always listened to what my body would tell me. I had a connection with my body and understood its language. I have always been a believer that your body speaks to you. I was lucky to have an understanding of my body. I knew something was up before I was told I had breast cancer. I was getting tired easily, which was not like me at all. I had blamed it on work. Whatever was going on, my body kept trying to tell me something was not aligned. Was I trying to fight this invader off and didn't even know what was going on inside of me? I just sensed something was wrong but couldn't pinpoint what it could be.

The weekend before my last radiation treatment, I made sure I had plans from Saturday morning until Sunday evening. I didn't even want to give myself any time to sit around and think about the last visit to come. I had already been wondering if I shouldn't stop the treatments while I was ahead. Saturday, one of my neighbors had invited everyone in our community to his backyard picnic. I walked down the street and saw he had a full yard already. I spotted someone I knew and sat with her until my girlfriend Claudia, who lived right across the street from me, arrived. I spent the rest of the afternoon with Claudia. After hours of conversation and laughs and after I had won a $30.00 gift certificate, I grabbed the centerpiece on our table and left for home. I wanted to save some energy for the next day.

Tenesha and I had plans for brunch that Sunday. I left it up to her to pick the spot. She picked a restaurant in Bridgeport by the ocean that served only organic food. I got up that Sunday morning feeling a bit under the weather. I called Tenesha to let her know I would need a few more hours to pull myself together. Our plans were changed to 2 P.M., rather than noon as originally planned. She was gracious enough to accommodate me. When I arrived at Tony and Tenesha's house, I had to wait for Tenesha to finish up. She had taken advantage of the delay and ran to the gym. I sat with Tony and chatted with him for a while. They lived across the street from the ocean. I could see the island Tony had told me about from their deck. When the tide is low, you can walk to the island. Tony would do his daily run to the island and back.

Jay, Tony's friend for over fifteen years, came to visit while I was still there. I hadn't seen Jay in years. He's one of the sweetest individuals I know. Jay has had a tough life and seemed to have lost his worth. I can see how hard it is for Jay to see his qualities. He has many of them, and my family loves him. I noticed he looked handsome in a different way today. Tony had told me Jay had a new girlfriend, and I couldn't help but think that she may have made the difference in the glow I was seeing in Jay as he sat across from me today.

Once Tenesha was done getting dressed, we took off to Blood Root in Bridgeport. It was a nice experience. The restaurant was quaint, and we helped ourselves. The day was gorgeous, and we chose to sit at an outside table. It felt as though we had been invited to someone's backyard. It didn't feel like a restaurant. The yard overlooked the ocean. The atmosphere seemed to be a bit feminist. Tenesha and I fit in just fine. Tenesha and I had so much to talk about, and it was nice to spend this time with her one-on-one, without Tony. It gave us a chance to get to know each other. I felt bad that since she and Tony had moved to Connecticut back in March I hadn't gotten the chance to spend the time I would have liked to with her. I had been going through my breast cancer ordeal since March and just didn't have the energy to do the things I would have liked to normally do with Tenesha. I finished my Spanish omelet and coffee, and we could see that the owners wanted to close up for the day. We could see a festival happening on the other side of the ocean and decided that would be our next destination. I couldn't tell you how we managed to find it, but we did. I parked the car and we walked up and down the boardwalk. There were plenty of vendors along the boardwalk, but we decided to spend most of our time by the dance floor. The cutest elderly man was on the floor dancing as if he were twenty years old. He wasn't dancing with anyone but having the best time of his life. He owned the dance floor that day.

I dropped Tenesha off a couple of hours later and headed home. I hadn't left Bailey alone for this long since I'd gotten him. I was starting to get nervous now. I rushed home only to find that Christina and Nick had been there and had tired him out for me. I forgot that Bailey had an extended family that loved him.

It turned out to be a great weekend for me, and I had only one more treatment left to go.

I noticed that the last week of radiation treatments had really drained me. I started to feel a dull pain in my chest when I took my walks with Bailey now. I promised myself I would not give in to this disease. I wasn't letting it take over my life. By the grace of God, I made it through my sixth and final week. My breast had gotten very swollen and sore. My nipples were super sensitive. I hadn't been sleeping very well by the sixth week. My right arm would turn numb during the night. I was starting to experience awful pain in my right hand. It would come only during the night. I was told that this was not a side effect of the radiation. I had no idea what this could be.

Monday came, and instead of being thrilled, I dreaded this last trip to the hospital. I wanted to call and cancel. It was so hard to bring myself to do this one more time. How foolish was this? I had gone through so much and now I wanted to give up? I had been using my radiagel faithfully. The hospital hands out radiagel for radiation patients for the "burn" area. It was a soothing gel that contained antibiotics. My skin was now a very deep brown. My skin had been tearing. My breast looked awful. It had undergone so much, which was now taking its toll. I stood in front of the mirror naked before I got dressed to go to the hospital for that last time. I looked at my good breast and wondered how I could have complained about myself in the past. I had never seemed to think I was pretty enough, sexy enough, or good enough. I would give anything to go back to the old me and be grateful for what God had blessed me with. God had given me so many blessings, and I had the nerve to complain instead of feel grateful. I learned a powerful lesson. I would not be less than anymore. I have become so much more, even with a tormented left breast.

I was on my way for what was my last ride to Midstate Hospital. I had mixed feelings. I was sad to say goodbye to the staff, yet I couldn't wait to put an end to this ordeal. As I expected, the staff was wonderful on my last day. I was given a healing metal with an angel on it from the radiation technicians. This would be something I would cherish. I do not want to ever forget this journey. We exchanged hugs and I made my way to the nurses' office before I left. She informed me that I would get worse before I started to heal. The radiation would continue to work on me for at least another two to three more weeks. I should expect to see my nipple tear, as had the skin under my breast and underarm. Damn—I was going to be leaving for Cape Cod that following Monday. I had no idea I would be getting worse. The week at the Cape was about healing, not getting worse.

I said goodbye to the staff one more time before my final exit. I promised I would bake some goodies for them when I returned from Cape Cod. They had always been smiling and pleasant every day and I wanted to acknowledge them and show my appreciation.

I finally left the building and looked back at the door I had walked into for what seemed to be an eternity. I was walking away from the door that read Cancer Center. I don't think I felt my feet touch the ground. I got into my car and I wanted to scream the words of Martin Luther King:
I AM FREE AT LAST — THANK GOD ---------- I AM FREE AT LAST

Life's Challenges

There are times in life you will feel challenged
You will question—have I not been through enough?
Have I not learned the lesson?

The week my radiation was completed was one of those
challenges for me
I decided to go back to a normal life thinking of everyone else but
myself

Again, did I not learn God gave me a second chance?
That I counted too?

Lyme disease visited me to remind me
Slow down Bruna and think of what is best for you

And most important of all
Listen to your spirit—it will never fail you

The week of my last radiation treatment was just terrible. At this point both my arms and hands were in pain. No one was able to give me a good reason why I was going through all of this. It had gotten so bad that when I tried to pick something up I couldn't even feel what I had in my hand. I would have a grip on something and drop it, as I had no control of my hands anymore. Could my Lyme disease have kicked in? Dr. Raxlen had a concern that this might happen and from the way I was feeling, my guess was that Lyme disease was my new visitor. My immune system was totally compromised. I had no idea what was happening to me. I felt as though I had become a target for anything these days. I had never been so vulnerable emotionally or physically in my life. I immediately called Dr. Raxlen and he squeezed me in for an appointment the Tuesday after my Cape Cod vacation. Keep in mind Dr. Raxlen is booked for months in advance. I had no doubt when I called he would see me. He's always been there for me for over fifteen years.

The nurse at the Cancer Center was right. I was getting worse each day. My breast and nipples were getting more sensitive as the days went on. It was a constant pain now. I still kept up with my walks with Bailey and tried to keep a normal lifestyle. I was not going to let my discomfort put a cramp in my life if I could help it. It took all my energy to keep up with a puppy like Bailey these days. I had plans to leave for the Cape that coming Sunday with Rich. I knew this was going to make or break us. I wanted to give it a last shot before I let go of a five-year relationship; or was it just a friendship? I wasn't sure how to look back at it. I didn't feel up to going to the Cape at all. I would have loved to call it off. Rich had already taken the week off from work. With that I felt I needed to go. I didn't feel it was fair to Rich, as he was so excited about doing his outdoor activities. I should have known how it was going to end up. We both knew I couldn't be out in the sun and we both knew I was bringing Bailey along. We both knew Bailey would need to be watched every minute of the day, as there was no crate to leave him in at the Cape. There would be no room in the car for the crate, so we knew it would to be left behind.

I was so drained and this week was going to be humid and in the 90s. Just what Bailey and I needed. I would have loved to leave Bailey home and get some real rest, but there was no one I could leave Bailey with. He was just over the top by now. He was also so attached to me, being with me constantly since the day I'd taken him home, that I didn't want to chance what would happen if I just up and left him in a kennel. There were times I wondered if I didn't make a mistake getting Bailey at this time in my life. There was nothing calm about this cute pup. From the time he awoke to the time he dropped at the end of the day, he was doing whatever he needed to get my attention and irritate the crap out of me. I couldn't get dressed without Bailey making a game out of it. It was tug-of-war time with my clothes each time I tried to get dressed. Of course, he seemed to always win. Then it became a game of "catch me if you can—it's the only way you'll get your clothes back from me." Bailey had taken over my couch as well. His hormones must have kicked in, as he would hump the pillows on my couch each morning and he would end the day in the same fashion. When I made myself breakfast, he would sit by me and bark until I gave him something. If I didn't share with him, he would sit there and bark through my whole meal. I gave up trying to read the morning paper. What had been an enjoyable time of my day for me became a nightmare with Bailey in my life. The walks were not fun anymore. It was so hot and humid outside now that Bailey would decide just several houses away that the walk was done. He became a mule. I would tug at him and he would not budge. Bailey wasn't getting the fact that although he was still a pup, he was getting too large for me to just pick up and carry home. When Bailey realized we were headed home, he became so happy he would start jumping and grabbing the leash and running, pulling me along with him. I started to feel foolish. The neighbors must have been at their window watching this comedy show every time I walked Bailey. Once we got through the front door after our walk, Bailey would start his "catch me if you can" game with anything he could grab and run with. This was all getting too old for me. I couldn't keep Bailey in his pen all day and I just didn't have the energy for his games anymore. I was stuck with this little monster twenty-four hours a day. I knew this was how it would be once we got to the Cape, only worse. I knew Rich wouldn't take part in Bailey's activities and there would be nowhere for me to put Bailey when I had enough of him. We were staying at one of my best friend's summer cottage at the Cape and I was going to have to be on Bailey more than ever so he did not destroy anything. Lord, I was not looking forward to this vacation at all.

This little angel of mine turned into a little demon. Erica took pictures of Bailey one day and she pointed out to me the two little horns he had in the pictures she took. When Bailey cocked his head down, his ears would fold in a way that would pull the skin in the front corner of his ears and make what looked like little demon horns. He had the markings on his back of wings of an angel and now he had the horns of a little demon child. I knew an exorcism was in order. There was just so much I could take, and these days Bailey was bringing me to tears.

I called a canine behavioral school in town and made my first appointment to teach this little monster manners. This started a whole new world of its own. I knew I wanted to enjoy my little companion, but I needed help controlling him first. I didn't have anyone in my life to share the responsibilities of this pup anymore. He had scared them all away. We didn't get to start the classes until we returned from the Cape, but I would come to realize it would not have made a difference anyway. Our first day at the behavioral school told me it was going to be a total waste. I would have to sit and talk to the trainer for over an hour and if Bailey and I were lucky we would squeeze ten minutes of training into the class. It wouldn't have been so bad if we talked about training my dog but oh no—I had to listen to stories of his family, his past, and best of all his part-time business. Five hundred dollars later and classes from hell, Bailey was no better than he was when we started. I actually felt sorry for Bailey. The trainer would have us sit in a warehouse that was at least 100 degrees with a fan blowing on us for an hour. He had one of his German shepards in a cage by the wall near where we would sit in the heat. I would forget his dog was in the cage until he would try to get out of the cage and scare the shit of me and Bailey. By the time he chose to give Bailey his ten-minute classes, Bailey was so hot and dehydrated that it was painful for me to watch him and even worse for Bailey. Every time Bailey would walk by the cage the trainer's dog was locked in, the dog would try to lunge for Bailey and scare the shit out of him. After a few of these classes, I stopped going. I didn't care how much money I lost. I felt this was a joke and a waste of my time. Fools like me kept this guy in business.

Everything about me was telling me not to head for Cape Cod this week. I thought I should just call and cancel or have Rich go alone without Bailey and me. Bailey alone would do me in, but I would come to find out how Rich would be tested that week. Maybe this is what the Cape vacation was all about. I decided to go with it even though I knew I should not.

I would always be the one to preach about listening to your gut, as it is always going to guide you in the right direction. Here I was turning my back on my gut feeling, my spirit telling me what I should be doing. I left for Cape Cod Sunday morning packed to the hilt with Rich and, yes, Bailey too.

Strength

When broken down emotionally and physically------------

Thank God we have that strength called spirit inside

This is a gift we were given while entering this life
It is our survival kit.

I couldn't believe I found myself on the way to the Cape and I really couldn't believe I found myself sitting in the back seat with Bailey as Rich was driving the three of us to Cape Cod. After a ride that seemed like an eternity and many pit stops for Bailey to relieve himself and to stretch, we finally arrived at the Cape. Tony and Tenesha were waiting for us in the large deck on the side of the house, loving the Cape and themselves together. I let Tony and Tenesha take the weekend to themselves so they could have some alone time before we got there with Bailey. They had just finished a lobster dinner and were enjoying the beautiful breeze that nighttime brings over the Cape. Shortly after we arrived, Tony and Tenesha left, as they had the long ride home and were up early for work the next day.

I felt wonderful that they'd had such a good time. They both said they wish they could stay longer. Not an hour into our stay, my four days from hell started. I would find myself with Bailey twenty-four hours a day. I had no pen for him, so it was me watching over Bailey all day and all night long. Bailey needed to feel or rather smell his new surroundings. He loved the smells of the rabbits and God knows what else that would stir around the property. It was brutally hot and very muggy and we had no air conditioner as we had back home. Bailey had no cement floor here as he did at home in his pen to lay his belly on to cool himself down. He couldn't find any vents shooting up cold air to rest over to cool off as he did at home. I could tell between his being in pain with his teething and the heat, not to mention his new surroundings, that he was off the wall. Or shall I say more off the wall than usual.

I kid you not when I say Bailey was literally attached to me for four days straight nonstop. Rich had no patience for this dog at all. I was not able to do anything with Rich, as I would have had to take Bailey, so I was very limited. The second day, we attempted to take Bailey to Providence Town. It was a scorcher, muggy, and neither Bailey nor I were doing well in the heat. Rich was truly tested that day. I did not find it enjoyable, and I know Rich wasn't doing well with the situation. After over two hours of walking in the heat and sun, we decided to leave and head back to the cottage. Evening came upon us and we had a double bed in the master bedroom. We were cramped to say the least, as Bailey decided to sleep with us. We had a fan in the window that faced the bed so it was blowing the night air on us. The three of us in one double bed lasted only one night. Rich and I had quarreled by the second night. I was getting upset that he was doing nothing to help out with Bailey and was able to shut us out completely to deal with our situation. On the third day of our vacation, Rich decided he would go out kayaking and returned with a hurt back. He had just recently gotten over a back injury and may have pushed it by staying out in the ocean for too long that day. He was probably staying away so he wouldn't have to deal with what was waiting for him back at the cottage. Bailey and a very weary me.

By Wednesday evening I was pushed to my limit. We had only been there three days, but I couldn't think of going through this one more day. I didn't even care to walk the beach with Bailey in the evenings, as I was fighting to keep him from going off the leash and running into the huge waves. I didn't think this would be an appropriate time to see how well my pup could swim. I had owned a black lab that was afraid of the water and, given the chance, would have drowned, and this left quite an impression on me. I knew I would not be able to rescue Bailey, as I couldn't swim and I didn't care to make my vacation any worse than it already was. I'm sure this was a foolish thought, but as much as I couldn't stand being with Bailey one minute longer, I knew I still loved the shit out of him and I couldn't live without him. He was becoming a child to me rather than a pup. The height of my days at the Cape was taking Bailey for walks. It was so hot and no fun at all. We just couldn't get away from the heat, and both Bailey and I were not dealing with this well at all.

I was hoping this vacation would have brought Rich and I closer as we were drifting apart very fast these days. I could see that this little puppy that Rich had decided to get with me became my pup. Rich didn't have the love and commitment it took to own a dog like Bailey. This is where knowing unconditional love comes in. I was starting to see things about Rich and realizing that if I chose to be with Rich, there would be many limitations in my life. The biggest was believing that Rich loved me. I could see that we were not able to communicate and that Rich was always on the defensive. I was finding out that you could not tell Rich he did something that hurt you, as I would get the same "I have nothing to apologize for and I did nothing wrong." He couldn't see past this. He couldn't see he was hurting me and didn't care to find out why or how or how we could both correct our differences. I was not feeling good at all by now. I was feeling the Lyme disease really kicking in. Emotionally I was drained from Bailey and my "discussions" with Rich. I told Rich I wanted to leave the next day, and we did just that. We packed up, cleaned up the cottage, and left for home. I just sat crying before we left. I couldn't hold it back one minute longer. I was so frustrated, tired, and upset. I decided to sit in the back seat with Bailey to make it easy on all of us for the ride home. As Bailey lay his head on my lap sleeping, I held back the tears. As much of a pain in the ass that this dog was, I knew he loved me unconditionally. I knew he had gone through so much with me in the short time I'd owned him. Bailey was there through all the times no one was for me through this journey. I reflected on my trip to the Cape. I tried to focus on some positives, and there were only two that I could think of.

My first thought was of the day we went to P town. As we were leaving P town, Rich and I stopped at my favorite shop. I was never able to go into this shop without walking out with something I loved. This shop is my reason for going to P town. This time I didn't see anything I could afford or that stood out saying "buy me, take me home." Just as I reached the door to exit the shop, there it was. It caught the corner of my eye as it sat alone on a table. My butterfly came back to me in an iron cast form. I had been looking for my butterfly I'd let go in the spring every day to see if it would find its way back to me. I had wished I could have kept it and framed it in a glass case to keep with me always, but my spirit would not allow me to hurt the beautiful creature. I believed this butterfly that caught my attention that day in the shop was a gift for me to fill that need for my butterfly that I had given back to nature. I would end up putting this butterfly on my dining room table for all to notice. Of course I knew no one would understand the full meaning of this butterfly, but it didn't matter. I did.

The second thought I was reflecting on was the last night of my Cape stay. I had a rose that came from a bush that Mary and Jesus had prayed at. I had carried this in my wallet for over twenty years. It was given to me years ago when I was going through a hard time. It became very special to me and I kept it in my wallet for all of these years. It never left me. I wanted to give a gift that was special to me to my ocean, the universe, the higher power—My God. I took a ride to the ocean the night before we left for home. I walked to the edge of the ocean. I thanked God and told him how grateful I was that he spared me and allowed me to catch my breast cancer at such an early stage. I wanted God to accept something that was special to me, as I was so thankful for his gift to me. My second chance. I delicately placed the rose into a wave and watched as it kept coming back to my feet. I asked that God please accept this as an offering for my appreciation of all I had learned in the last four short months. I placed the rose back into the next wave and the wave took it out to sea. When I felt it was accepted, I looked out into the horizon of the sky letting daylight go to evening and held that picture in my mind as I thanked God for all he had done for me and would continue to bring into my life. I realized that my breast cancer was a journey of change and second chances. I had brought this crazy loving dog into my life and would have endless years of love and companionship with Bailey. I would enjoy my children and their lives more as I would be enjoying my life more. I would look at my life much differently than I had been. As broken as I looked and felt, there was that pilot light still inside of me stronger than ever. God's light, my gift.

With these thoughts, I looked down at Bailey sleeping with his head on my lap. I stroked Bailey's head and looked up at Rich driving us and I had to smile as I wondered how silly this must look to people driving by us. I felt like Miss Daisy, and Rich was my driver. The smile slowly left me as I realized I would soon be ending my relationship with Rich altogether. It would be such a shame, as we had so much in common—our likes and dislikes, the way we thought of nature and spirit in life. I had thought he understood me when I felt things that most individuals in my life would call me crazy for. There was a very deep friendship bond. Would I be able to keep this friendship with this man after we disconnected? I felt he was not happy with me, as he could not love me as a woman or a partner. I was frustrating him now, as I needed more since my breast cancer journey. I found life to be too short not to have someone to share life with. Rich didn't want this. He was perfectly content with what we had and didn't need me to make waves. Rich had introduced so much into my life that I would not have experienced or known if I had not had these past years with him. I suppose there is a reason why people come into our lives. I also know that we have to be smart enough to let them go when it's time.

My feeling was that Rich was still a child looking for fun in life and that in the last four months I grew up too fast for him.

Resilience

When we feel there is no more to give
When we feel there is no more to gain
When we feel we are on the brink of giving up

Our spirit is equipped to reach for our inner strength
To rescue us

If you listen it will give you instructions
If you turn away and choose not to listen
It will make the experience grueling but
In the long run you will end up with the same answer

Your spirit will protect you
However it needs to

It will happen in a way that you will choose to listen to the answer
Life will bring you around and it will be your choice
You will get the answer one way or other.

We finally made it home from the Cape. I looked wired, literally. I saw that both Erica and Christina were home. I got out of the car and brought Bailey inside while I unpacked Rich's car so he could leave and get home as well. Of course Christina and Erica went nuts when they saw Bailey. Four days away from this adorable pup!!!! If only they knew what I had just gone through.

Christina and Erica decided they were going shopping, so it was Bailey and me again. I unpacked, did some laundry, and watered my garden, as it was half dead by the time I got home. This time I had a pen to leave Bailey in. I needed that time of separation badly. I put Bailey in his pen and he seemed very content. His toys were all around him and he went right over to his bed and fell into it. Bailey was quiet, so he must have needed the time away from me just as much as I needed the time away from him. I was trying to bring my flowers and plants around, as the heat had taken its toll on them. As I finished and was putting the hose away, I felt ready to just collapse in my front lawn. Right about this time, Christina and Erica pulled into the driveway after their little shopping spree. They stood there looking at me and laughing hysterically. I was dead at this point. My hair by this time was in a full-blown fro and the distress on my face was indescribable. You can't imagine how I felt and looked at that point. I wanted to find a hole to crawl into and just stay there for a while until I got my bearings again. I wanted some quiet time and peace, which I knew was now impossible in my life. No way was Bailey going to allow me to have any of that.

Once showered and somewhat relaxed, I sat on my back deck. It was early evening, and the sunlight was golden that time of day. I thought about my last five years with Rich. I realized I had done it again. I had created a man in my mind that never existed. How many times was I going to allow this to happen to me in my life? Would my breast cancer journey keep things real from now on? As the weeks went by, I would see Rich less and less. I thought I couldn't feel any more alone than I had, but life managed to throw another punch at me. I knew I had to stop seeing Rich altogether but was so afraid to end it completely. I wasn't on my feet from breast cancer just yet. Was this really the best time to cut the ties altogether? But then was Rich really in my life anyway?

It wasn't until I had my appointment with Dr. Raxlen that Tuesday for my Lyme disease that I knew what I had to do. Dr. Raxlen and I discussed my situation concerning Rich. I could see by the end of the conversation with Dr. Raxlen that Rich had a completely separate life from me. He never let me into his space at all. He would share my world but I was kept away from his. Did I not think enough of myself that I allowed this to go on for five years? I did finally get the courage to end it. Whether we would keep somewhat of a friendship remained to be seen, but the relationship part was finally done. We were both free from each other.

I couldn't wait to get back to work and throw myself into something to take up my life now. My days were idle with nothing to do but think and get my strength back. I was on medication for my Lyme disease and would be off from work for several more weeks to give the medication time to kick in while I rested. Bailey was getting worse rather than better. He tested me all day long. He just wanted my attention constantly while I was home. He wanted to play the game of "catch me if you can" all day long. He would grab things and expect me to run around the house grabbing it back from him. When I no longer cared what he had in his mouth, he decided he would make me care. He seemed to know what I didn't want broken and was now taking off with those special items so I would have to run after him and take them back. In the evening he seemed to become possessed with some demon force. He would have these play sessions with us, but was still nipping. Well, now he was five months old and his teeth were not just baby teeth anymore. They were starting to hurt. The thought of giving Bailey up to another family crossed my mind these days. Was it fair to this dog to keep him? Would I ever get the energy I once had? He needed constant exercise and I had no idea where I was headed with my health or my life. Bailey was my cancer dog. I'd grown to love him. I could see I was his life. Besides, who would tolerate this monster as I did? There had to be a reason Bailey was in my life. I needed to give us a chance. I was not in any sort of normal space in my life. There was no way I could give this dog to anyone. I would die without him. He had become my life. I'm sure he would get better as he got older. I couldn't give one more thing up in my life right now anyway.

When Bailey had his normal moments, he was absolutely gorgeous. I would just admire him as we sat outside in the warm summer sun. We both enjoyed that time together. I could see the bond we had together. He loved me. He truly loved me. He would not go to sleep at night unless he was in my bed and bumped right up against my legs. He'd let out a huge sigh and then fall asleep. As if now everything was perfect for us. I would have to admit how comforting this was for me these days as well. Each day after our walks, we would sit on the grass and enjoy the warm sun beating down on us. Bailey loved to sprawl out so that the warm grass caressed his belly. Our favorite spot was by the butterfly bush next to my house, as it got the most sun during the day. By this time it was July and I had stopped waiting for my butterfly that I let go back in May to find its way home to me. It was off on its own journey and I would not have the pleasure to meet up with it again. I supposed it had served its purpose for me and moved on.

Bailey loved to try to go after the small white butterflies that were all around us. They would surround the butterfly bush and would flutter around us each time we sat by it. We would see the tiger swallowtail butterflies and the monarch butterflies, but my spicebush never showed. They would allow me to pet them and lift them on my finger. I suppose we had become friends. I got to know them each. There was always a flaw or some marking that made them unique. Like the tiger swallowtail that had an injured wing and always landed on me as if to just say "hi." The energy of the butterflies just lifted my spirits and was so healing for me.

One particular afternoon after one of our walks, as usual, Bailey and I sat by the bush. A beautiful butterfly flew right up to Bailey and fluttered around his head. It then turned to me and fluttered around me. I thought to myself, "Here's a new butterfly that acts as though we're best friends." It finally landed on my butterfly bush next to us. I wanted to touch this butterfly and see if I could lift it on my fingers as I did my other butterflies. I stood staring at this butterfly and became teary eyed. I lifted it on my finger and it sat there for the longest time. I then placed it back on the bush and stroked its wings. It sat there and allowed me to stoke its wings for as long as I liked. It was a spicebush swallowtail butterfly with the identical colors as the one I'd released just before my radiation treatments back in May. Could it be????? I would never really know, but it became a regular visitor to my butterfly bush. When I would have a down day, I noticed it would visit. I'd like to think it was another sign of God telling me to stay strong and never stop believing.

I had three more weeks to go before I got back to work. I was feeling better from the Lyme disease and the effects of the radiation. Each day was better for me. I was starting to see signs of Bruna returning once again. I started up my vitamin C IV drips to get some strength back and jump-start my immune system. I tried to get back to the gym but just wasn't ready for my normal routine just yet. It would come soon enough.

The next three weeks came and went in a blink of an eye. The first week I returned back to work, Bailey turned six months old. It was time to get my pup neutered. I thought this might help with his behavior, but I was kidding myself. He did eventually stop humping the sofa pillows, but that's about all it did. By this time my sofa needed to be thrown out. I'll spare the description. Let's just say my new couch is very nice and we've managed to keep it that way. I had been nervous about leaving Bailey at the vet overnight. This was the very first time he had gone without me since I'd gotten him. I think mom was more upset than the pup. We woke up early the morning of his operation and went for our regular walk. He jumped into the front seat of the car so excited. Yes Bailey, we're going for a ride. Little did he know what was about to happen to him. Once at the vet we went in, a nurse came to get him, and neither Bailey nor I knew what happened and he was gone into another room. I got into my car and felt terrible. I'm sure Bailey realized by then that I wasn't there and was going nuts. To top it off, he would be caged until I picked him up tomorrow. That evening as I lay in bed without my buddy, a huge thunderstorm rolled in. It was the hottest night of the summer, and all I thought was, "What if the electricity is lost at the vet?" No air, no light, and these huge cracks of thunder. I felt scared for Bailey. The vet told me I could pick Bailey up at noon the next day. I had a meeting in the office that would run until noon the next day and wouldn't be able to pick him up until the afternoon. I felt awful that I couldn't get him in the morning. I finally got out of my meeting at exactly noon and raced to the vet to pick up my "baby." I couldn't walk fast enough to the reception desk at the vet to ask them to get Bailey for me. While waiting for my pup, I found out the electricity had gone out overnight. Poor Bailey, neutered, hot, in pain and thunder. What a first-time experience he had away from me. I was told to keep Bailey still. No running or jumping. Were they kidding me? Once I got Bailey home and he saw his familiar surroundings, he ran around for thirty minutes straight. Up and down the stairs, around the house. I was dizzy watching him. They had not given me any meds for this dog, and I couldn't believe he could run around like this. Was he feeling no pain? He was so swollen I hurt for him, and here he was like a maniac running around the house. I couldn't even catch him to keep him still. He would look at me with that "No way are you coming near me" look. But then this was Bailey; could I expect anything less than this behavior?

I had introduced Bailey to his dog walker the week prior to my starting back at work. I did this more for her benefit than Bailey's. I wanted Louise, Bailey new dog walker, to know what she was getting herself into. I wanted to be sure on the days I could not be home and on the road that Bailey got exercised and some attention midday. Louise seemed to do fine with Bailey, even though he was now sixty-five pounds and had a mind of his own while on walks. It was hard for both Bailey and me to go through the separation. We had been attached at the hip for four months. I tried to work at home a couple of days a week, but I needed to be out on the road to make a living for us. I realized it wasn't just Bailey that couldn't live without me—I couldn't live without this little monster in my life either.

Grieving

As the days went by and I began to heal I started to feel the grief
All of a sudden I allowed myself to grieve the loss of my
marriage
I allowed myself to cry and hurt over the divorce
I came to realize I never did this
I had swallowed the hurt and never allowed myself to feel the
pain
I turned it all to anger and let it manifest in me—how could I find
happiness like this?

In my days of healing from my cancer journey I began to heal
from life

I grieved my relationship with my older brother. I allowed myself
to accept the fact that he was no longer in my life.
I felt this was his choice. I have learned to respect the decision he
has made and move on with my life without the need of my older
brother being a part of my life.
He meant the world to me growing up and it was such a grief to
have to let go of this.

I have accepted my ex husband as a friend. I am hopeful he will
come to terms with this as well. I will always love him as family.
He was family for twenty-seven years of my life and this is very
difficult for me to just wipe away as if it never existed.

I have accepted my breast cancer
I have accepted my Lyme disease
I will not focus on either
I choose to help others not as blessed as I have been

I realize I am not solo in my life
I have myself and my children (and of course Bailey)
There are many that do not have that much. I am grateful for all I
have today

I will accept whatever God sends me with gratitude
I hope that for the rest of my journey I am all I was meant to be

I hope I leave my children proud of me. If I accomplish just that
my life will have been well worth it

By my third week back to work, I was tackling it with a vengeance. I had accumulated so many bills I needed to make my sales to pay these debts off. It was rather scary, as prior to my cancer episode I was doing okay in my financial affairs. How fast one can tumble down in just four months. But then those had been no ordinary four months either. Back at work, there were changes in management I was going to have to deal with. I shortly found out that no one had a clue what they were doing in this new organization. It seemed as though individuals were being assigned to positions in the company they had no business being in. It didn't take long for me to figure out I had walked into the same mess I'd stepped out of before I'd gone out for short-term leave. It might have even gotten worse.

I was still going for my weekly vitamin C IV drips, but within the first month of my return to the office I had become so exhausted. I found myself canceling my IV drips and doctor appointments, as I had so much work to do when I got back to the office, I couldn't keep up. I was beginning to work nights and weekends and was slowly starting to fall back into my old patterns once again. I didn't find it so bad at the beginning of the week, but by Friday I felt like a wet rag. The weekends were really hard for me. I was seeing everyone go out and having a great time as I sat home alone with Bailey driving me nuts. I guess I was lucky to have Bailey. He gave me some company so that I wasn't feeling as alone as I could have been. I found myself going grocery shopping on Saturday night just so I could get out of the house. I was realizing how sad my life had become. I was forgetting how lucky I was and all the things I had planned to do. Now I was sitting trying to figure out how I would get the energy to do them all.

I found myself so alone one night that I signed myself up for a free trial on one of the dating sites on the Internet. I found out very soon in this game that this was not for me. If there was supposed to be someone in my life, I would find him and it would not be on a dating site because I was feeling sorry for myself on a Saturday night.

I would speak to Rich on occasion. He seemed to miss me at first, but as time went on I was seeing him sliding back into a "lone wolf" pattern that seemed to reside deep inside of him. I had no doubt that in the very near future he would speak of me as a dear friend that used to be in his life. We have people that come into our lives for a reason. We touch each other's lives for a reason. I hope my part was a positive experience for Rich and I will always wish him happiness.

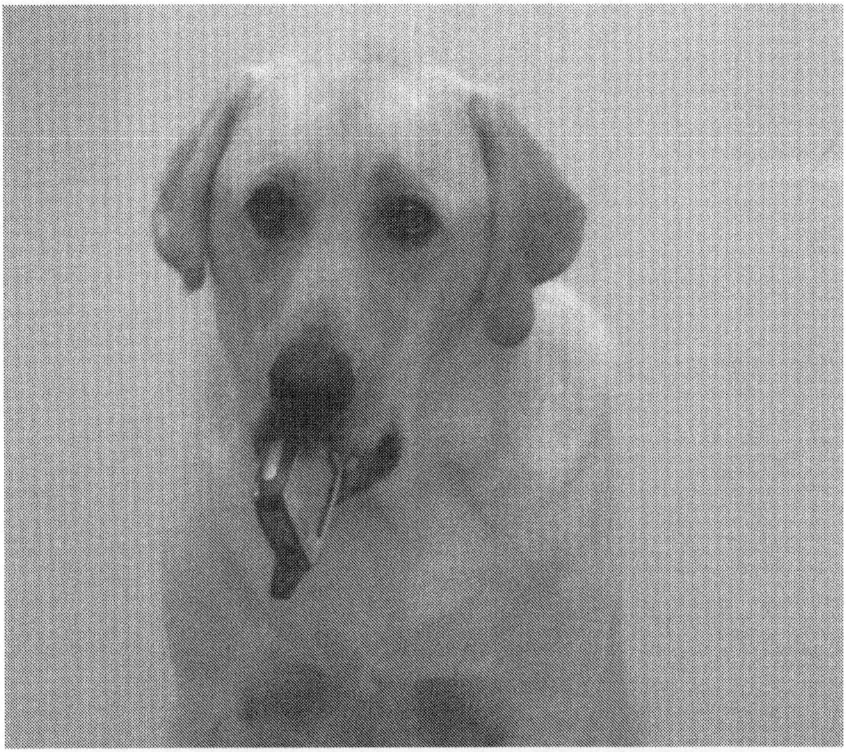

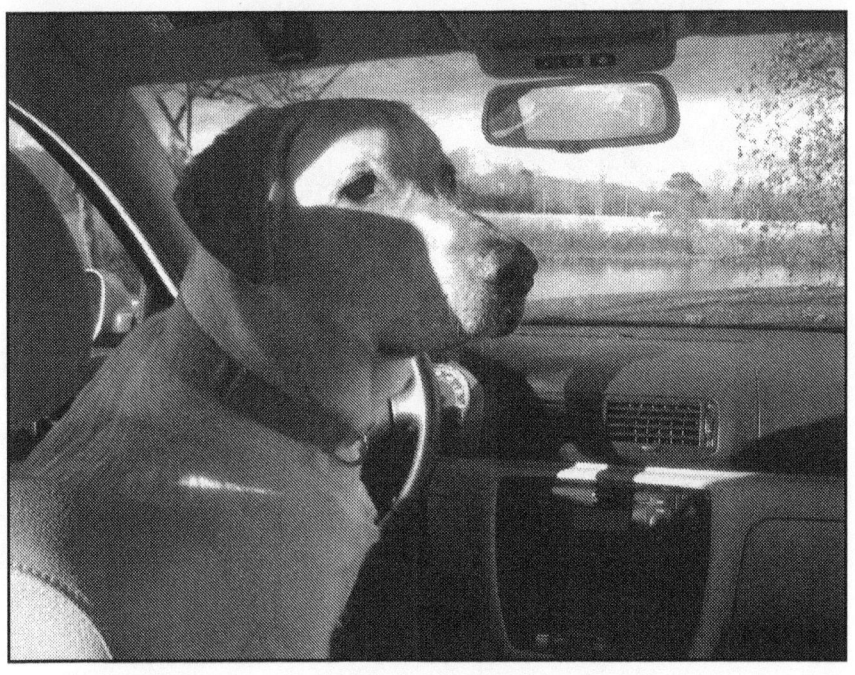

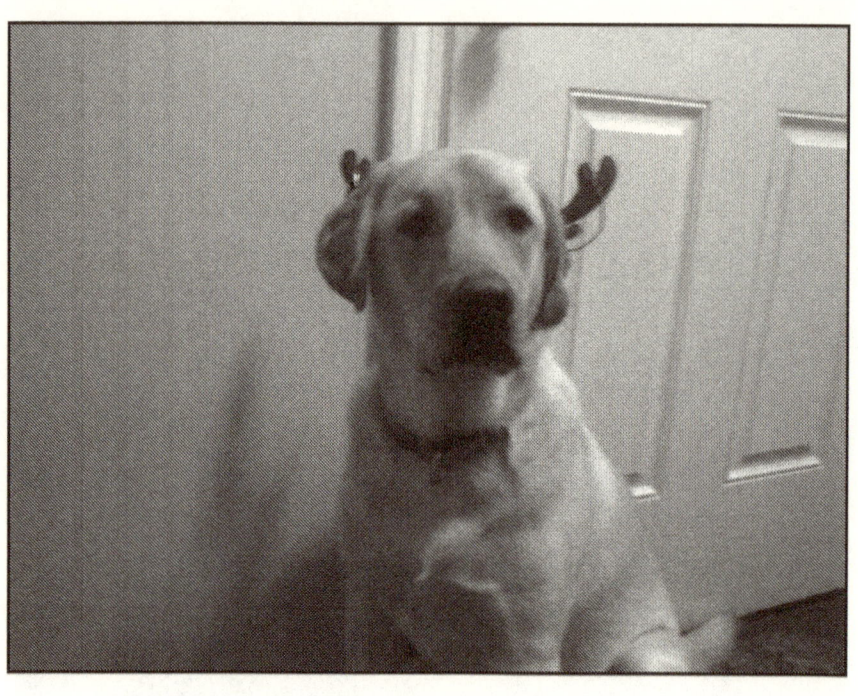

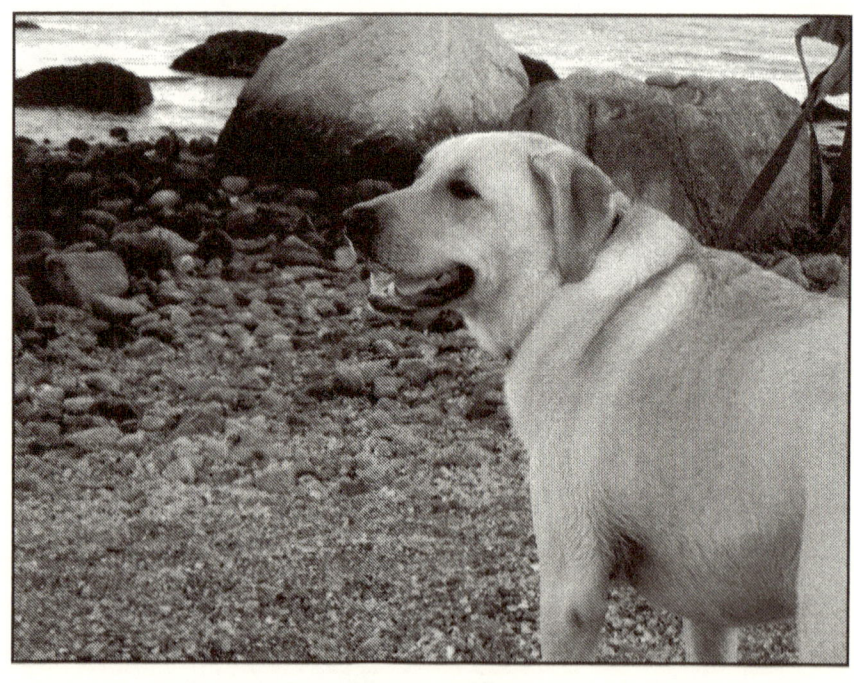

Nothing Seems To Remain The Same

As the Buddhists say
Nothing ever remains the same.

One would like to think that when you are in a perfect time in
your life
When you feel you have been blessed
When you think you have been found
When you think you finally got it

Poof
Right in your face

Time walks in and you realize how very mortal you are
This world has trained us into being earthly soldiers

We have been brainwashed or brain dead—take your pick
We pick up where we left off as it is second nature to us

Once thrown back into the mortal world
We seem to take off where we left off

Shame on us

A whole year flew by me. It was now one year ago that I had received my call letting me know that I had breast cancer.

Throwing myself back into work with a vengeance just about killed me. I wanted so much to be successful. When I realized that the government accounts were just not working for me and that no one was going to step forward and give me a break but in fact the opposite, try to break me, I took a Healthcare Rep position. An opening for the Healthcare territory in the Hartford area became available and I raised my hand. Once again being told one thing and given another. As time went on, I realized that I was seeing too many familiar things on this team. I realized the management wanted the numbers, and there was no type of fairness or respect for one another. It was so cutthroat, and I slowly became so disgusted with the whole thing. I loved sales, but I could not compromise myself, as so many were doing. I lost respect for my manager, for many of my team members, and for the office in general. The energy was exhausting, and I found myself hating to go into the office. How could these people waste so much energy being fake to one another? How did they trust one another, or did they not have an integrity at all? Did they know what it was?

Fall went by and I still hung in there. Winter was horrible. It was so hard at this point. I was starting to lose touch with my friends again. I was beginning to see my children less and less. I was truly falling back into the same pattern. Rich and I would talk, but weeks went by before we would even see each other briefly for a few minutes at a time. We both tried to keep the friendship going, but I really felt that Rich was trying to prove that he wasn't falling back into his old patterns. I'm not sure if it was for his sake or mine. I do know it seemed very hard for him to do.

Christmastime was not a real happy one for me that year. I felt alone, and my sister topped it off for me. My sister and her family planned to have Christmas dinner with me and my children, so I did have a fun day to look forward to. Several days before Christmas, my sister called to tell me she was no longer coming over Christmas day. At first she tried hard to not give me a reason why, but I did finally pry it out of her. She informed me that she had gotten another offer for Christmas day and would be going there instead. When she told me where she was going, it just devastated me. My older brother had asked her and her family over, and I was just brushed aside. After my phone conversation with my sister, I grabbed Bailey and we went for a long walk in the cold. I needed to have a good cry and did not want anyone to see me. I felt numb. I couldn't even feel how cold it was, nor did I see how dark it had become. I just kept walking. This was the first Christmas after my breast cancer episode. How could anyone hurt me like this? My family kept showing me time and time again how insignificant I truly was to them. At this point, I had to accept the way my family had become, as nothing that my family did penetrated me in any way anymore. I have become so numb to them. I share nothing with them. I have the understanding that they do not care what happens to me, so I keep to myself. I have learned the hard way. Yes, I do have my children but do not want to give them the burden of a parent alone and sometimes scared. They have enough going on in their lives at this time. I will not add burden to them. I would just love to have one person to call and share everything with. One person that I know would be there for me. Someone to do things with. I have been staying home every weekend for months now. My confidence is going down. Between feeling unsuccessful at work and feeling unloved—how do I keep it together?

There was one constant in my life every day through the breast cancer journey and still ongoing.

Bailey, my buddy.

I had been taking Bailey to doggie day care. I now started to take Bailey to doggie care three to four times a week, as it worked out well for me. Those days were wonderful. I would pick him up and he just slept until the next morning. I didn't have to worry about him being alone all day long while I was gone. The days he did not go were another story. Bailey was still our little bandit. He was constantly stealing everything that meant anything to Erica and me. He managed to destroy many things, including my $350 pair of designer glasses. One night I couldn't find Bailey, as he was so quiet. I looked up at the top of the stairs and saw him so handsome sitting so proud looking at me as if to say, "What's the problem, mom? Look how good I am. Come love me." I did. I sat next to him and gave him a hug and kisses and then saw something sticking out of his mouth. It was green and stiff. I now saw my lenses in pieces on the rug. I pulled my frames out of his mouth. "I can't do this anymore. There is something wrong with this dog and I can't deal with it anymore." I sat and cried.

I wasn't making the money I needed at work in sales. I couldn't afford to buy another pair of glasses. Erica gave me her old pair to wear. They were red with rhinestones around the frame. I tried them on and could make things out in the distance but could not see well out of them. Plus: RED WITH RHINESTONES!! Looked great on Erica - . but not on me—*Saturday Night Live* would have done a skit on me wearing these glasses. One ringy dingy—need I say more?

I would run out of toilet paper, kleenex, and paper towels by midweek. Thank you, Bailey. These seemed to be his favorite "come get me" toys. My hair brushes had teeth marks on the handles. I'm not sure what bills I received and should pay and what bills Bailey ate on me. If Erica or I turned our back on food, Bailey was tall enough to swat anything off the counter and grab it off the floor before we could get to him. By the time we caught Bailey, he was digesting whatever he'd grabbed. Food or not, it went down. My vet bills were ridiculous at this point. I was jacking up my Mastercard with Bailey issues. I could not quite understand how ten minutes after he'd traumatized me, I would go over to him and be capable of loving him and have a knowing that no matter what he did, I could not live without him. He was my constant. Even if it was a constant pain in the ass, he was constant. He never let me down. I knew he would drive me crazy every day of my life and he came through for me. I also knew that there was such a love for me from Bailey. I was what he lived to see and be with every day. I was his friend. He could count on me being there no matter what he did. He could count on me loving him no matter what he did. I felt the same about Bailey. He made my life these days. Sometimes good and sometimes really bad. Nothing else mattered as long as my buddy Bailey was there for me.

Denial

Isn't it funny how we as humans think we have it all together?
We admit we have had trauma and we think we learned the lesson

How many of us like myself go right back into old habits and
patterns once the trauma is over?
My denial continued
While going through my breast cancer experience, I was going
to conquer the world when I was back on my feet. I was going to
volunteer, help other woman—on and on

Who was I kidding? I barely had enough energy to take care of
myself and get through the week at work

God must have been watching me like the good father he is and
was waiting for me to fall on my face again. "Will this child of
mine ever learn?"

Not yet father, but soon -------------

As the days and weeks and months went by, I became more and more exhausted. I threw myself back into life as if I had not undergone a thing. It was as though I'd had a tooth pulled. Kind of like -----childbirth. I truly forgot the whole experience. Everything I planned on doing, including finishing my book, was on hold. Work was taking all the energy I had out of me. I had started to have problems with my arms and hands after my radiation treatments. The arms finally got better, but my hands continued to become worse every day. I was told it was not the radiation, but I'll never buy that one. I had been getting cortisone shots to relieve the pain in my hands, as I did not want to take the time out for surgery. I would get cortisone shot in the thumb joint and the base of the middle finger of both hands. I had carpal tunnel and trigger finger on both hands. Thank God we had a rather mild winter. Each time we had snow fall and I would go out and shovel, I was in the doc's office for my cortisone shots days later. The doc knew when he saw me just what to do.

The environment at work had become so stressful; my team members were walking around like zombies. One of my coworkers was getting chest pains, and this made me take a good look at my surroundings. It was looking dim for most of us in this corporation. I hated it more and more every day. The demands were ridiculous. Management truly did not know what the hell they were doing. Work was like a scene out of the Three Stooges. Who's on first, what's on second, I don't know, who's on third—no one knew what they were doing, nor did they have any direction. It was coming from top-level management down to bottom-level management. I was so nervous working for this corporation; I actually transferred out my company stocks.

My experience with Bailey and doggie day care were worrying me these days. It was bad enough that our first experience with doggie day care had been a nightmare, but now the dog care I had found and liked was not making Bailey happy and he was starting to let me know. It had worked out for months and now it wasn't looking good for Bailey. I hated to go back to the dog walker, as Bailey would be alone all day except for the half hour the dog walker came to visit him.

The first doggie day care I had brought Bailey to lasted all of two days. We didn't even get to finish our three-day trial. The "teacher" was waiting for me the second day I came to pick Bailey up. "Never again" I was told. I guess Bailey sat in front of this particular teacher and barked at her all afternoon. She had a migraine by the time I picked him up. She could not get him to stop barking at her. When she saw me there to pick Bailey up, she couldn't let him out of the play area for me fast enough. He wanted out so bad that he ran right by me to the front store area. Now that was the play space Bailey was looking for. It was a good thing they didn't charge me for the toys Bailey decided were his. He seemed to think he was on a shopping spree and I would get him anything he could grab in two minutes. I finally got Bailey in the car. I just looked at him. He gave me those "what's the problem? I'm never going there again, ma" looks. "Bailey, what am I going to do now? I can't leave you alone home all day. Do you want to stay in your pen until I get home?" Bailey could have cared less. He just wanted to go home.

I checked the Web and found another doggie day care. This one was a training school as well. Perfect!! I think Bailey thought after the first shot at doggie day, I would let it go. To his surprise I dropped him off at his second doggie day care. This one was very different from the first. I liked it much better. They were just starting up the doggie day care area, and there were only three dogs in this huge warehouse. This is the one we decided on. Bailey did fine considering. I mean fine in that they decided he could stay. The owners were absolute dolls. They had to Bailey-proof the whole warehouse. Bailey somehow managed to open all the doors in the warehouse and let himself out. He would open the bathroom door as well. They did work with Bailey, and he seemed to be managed by the group. The best part of this was picking Bailey up knowing that he was so wiped out, he would sleep. Now this was how a dog should be. I wasn't able to take him every day, as it was quite expensive. The days I was on the road all day he would be dropped off. The days I worked from home, he stayed home with me.

This worked out well for several months. Eventually Bailey developed separation anxiety. I was called quite often to pick Bailey up, as he was vomiting and had diarrhea quite frequently. After weeks of this, the owner of the doggie day care decided I should have Bailey checked out thoroughly by the vet before I brought him back again. Five hundred dollars later, I was told he missed me, and that was his problem. Good Lord, Why me??? I am fifty-five years old. The last thing I needed was another child. I'd been scared to death that there was a serious problem, but the vet assured me that all Bailey had was separation anxiety. Should I feel good that there is one soul that absolutely needs me in this world? I drove Bailey home after the visit to the vet and we sat on the front porch. He was on the warm pavement in front of my front steps, the sun shining on him. He looked at me with those big brown beautiful eyes. I could just tell what he wanted to say to me: "I can't help it if I love you that much, mom." A few tears ran down my face, and I had to hug him and tell him that's okay. We'll figure something out. I grabbed his head and looked into his eyes and said, "It's you and me, buddy. You know I can't live without you. You're here to stay no matter what." Bailey licked me and without a word or bark we knew we had a very special love for each other. After all—he was my cancer dog. He'd gotten me through it all in his own way.

This was the first time I took a look at how crazy my life was getting. Was Bailey telling me to slow down? All I did was work these days. The long days turned into long nights as well. This overflowed into the weekends. I had lost touch with my life again. Bailey was the only one that was calling my attention to it.

It's really not funny how things work out sometimes. After shoveling the driveway with the last snowfall we had that winter, I could barely move my right hand. After a month of being in pain, I made an appointment to see an orthopedic doctor. All I wanted was cortisone shot again to relieve the pain. The doctor would not allow me to have any more cortisone shots. I had reached my limit. With that, I found myself working from home more often, as I could not carry my laptop and case with my right hand in constant pain. This was working out for Bailey.

I was slowly starting to become so exhausted that I cried at the drop of a hat. The unfairness in the office was so obvious by now that it was in my face and I could not turn my head any longer. It was so bad that when the doctor told me I could no longer put off surgery on my hand, I was thrilled. I didn't care what I needed to do, but I needed a break from the office and the people in it. This also solved my problem with Bailey for a while. I would be on short-term disability and he would have me all day to himself. It was as though he'd wished this on me. It didn't matter how it all happened; I was thrilled I was getting away from the poison in my office. I could now reconnect with myself again and get moving on the things that were so important to me. The things I just couldn't find the time to do or get started because of the demands at work.

Here it was again. A year later and I was being sat still again. How many times would I have to be brought here before I listened and got it? I became so busy that I couldn't hear God once again. I wasn't listening again. Well, I was getting another chance. AGAIN

My Poor Body

My mom and dad managed to go through seventy-five years of their lives without any incisions in their bodies. How do the old Italians do that? Do they ignore any wrong in their bodies? Do they shut themselves off to pain? Have we become the weak generation? The generation that runs to the doctor because we may not be able to do our everyday routine without pain or discomfort?

My parents have passed on and every day I find there is a question I need to ask them. I never took the time as I was growing up. Too much fun to be had. I never had the time when I married, as I was too busy with household chores and raising children.

I am still now. I would give anything to have my dad come over this morning. I would make him his espresso. Grounds packed down so it would be very strong. We could sit on my deck and converse as we have so many times in my life. Only this time I have a ton of questions and this time I would finally listen to him.

What I would give for that moment in time

Love you papa

One year later and I found myself at Midstate Medical Hospital once again. This time it was no big deal. No cancer to deal with. I just had my hand cut in three different places. This was a piece of cake.

Erica had taken the time off from work to bring me once again. I would be home by noon. Once the surgery had been done, I was wheeled back to my room. I spotted my street clothes on the chair next to me. I wasn't about to wait for any nurse to give me permission to get dressed. I got up and threw my clothes on, as I couldn't wait to get the hell out of the hospital. It was starting to turn into a home away from home. I have no idea how I managed to get dressed with my hand just operated on. I suppose the drugs were doing their job for me. I finally got wheeled out of the hospital but I was not about to leave just yet. I saw there was a Dunkin Donuts on my way out and Erica had to get me my large cream-only coffee. Erica stopped to pick up my painkillers on the way home. She got me settled and made sure I had everything before she left for work. I assured her I was fine.

Not thirty minutes after Erica had left for work, I realized what I would be going through for the next month. The pain was starting to set in, and I remembered the doctor telling me to get the painkillers in me as soon as I got home. Okay, great. The pills were in one of the twist and hold-down containers. I have one good left hand. Great, how would I do this? I tried to hold the pill container between my knees and twist and hold down. The container went flying across the room several times. The only option I had was to smash the container to pieces.

Next I got hungry. I wanted a bagel. There it was on the counter. Now how do I cut it in half? It won't fit in the toaster whole. I held down the bagel with my right elbow and tried to cut with my left hand. I couldn't master this either. I almost sliced my elbow off.

My hair—oh you should have seen my hair for the first three weeks. There was no way I could blow-dry my hair and it went wild. I have very curly, kinky hair. What a sight. I'm sure no one would have taken notice if I had been in NYC, but I was in Wallyworld. If you wore too much makeup, you became a freak, and the whole town would be talking. I knew eventually the story, completely distorted at this time, would get back to someone in my family. I was already the black sheep, and I hadn't told anyone in my family I was getting my hand done. Lord only knows the story that would go on about me. I needed bandages one day, as I ran out of dressings for my hand. I put myself together as best I could and ran into Stop and Shop, our local grocery store. The stares I got!! My point was made. I was waiting for the call asking me if I'd joined a hippy commune, the way I looked. I looked like a fifty-five-year-old hippy that had not quite moved on. Still looking to follow the Grateful Dead.

Around the second week into this crap, I lost it. Bagels were flung to the walls of my kitchen. I was not eating well, as I couldn't make anything. Try not using your dominant hand for a month. Trust me when I tell you it will break you. I realized I could do nothing, even though I fought it and tried to anyway. I couldn't finish my book, as I could not type. I couldn't leave the house, as I would scare people. Bailey and my children were the only ones I would allow to see me like this. There would be no judgments made. They loved me and I knew it. Any way and in any package I came.

This did give me a chance to think. When you are still, you will find that the pain you have held inside does start to surface. Once again I realized God was speaking to me. Once again I realized I was listening. Through all of what I had gone through in this past year, I had not gone to one support group, nor had I gotten any counseling for my breast cancer or any of the pain I was trying to separate myself from in my life. God had a plan for me. I was going back to the journey I had not quite completed one year ago. It started to sink in. Oh trust me; I didn't get it right away.

I became bored not doing anything during the first month of my hand surgery. I signed up for another dating site. I realized all too quickly that this was just not a fit for me. I had gone from a marriage that I'd allowed to make me feel less than a woman to a five-year relationship that had made me feel even less of a woman than my marriage. I had not experienced anyone in my life to make me feel special.

There was no way anyone I was getting "winks" from on a dating site was going to do it for me. I did not want to make another mistake. At this point I was truly starting to think I was attracted to men who would treat me less than. I had to find out what was wrong with me.

My children and Bailey were all that mattered to me in life. There was a missing link for me, though. I could use a man that truly loved me in my life. I was now seeing that I needed to get help to clear the space for that person to come into my life. I thought I could keep Rich as a friend but started to realize that Rich was never really ever there. That can become draining after a while. I had to completely let go of Rich. I gave him permission out loud to be with other woman. I felt he had been there for a while now, but I needed to hear myself give him permission.

I was trying very hard to be friends with my ex. In trying to do so, I realized how much he had moved on. Once again, feeling less than. Was anyone going to ever love me in a way that would make me actually feel loved? The way the old-timers loved? I still believe there is one person out there that will be a soul mate. That will get me and love me so much that no one else could exist for him. Am I living a fairy tale? Will I ever find this person after breast cancer and one scarred breast?

I called the "Y-Me" breast cancer hotline. This was my first step toward getting help. After a conversation with the woman on the hotline, I realized I needed to speak to someone who had gone through what I had gone through—that I can and should believe there are men who truly can love me and make me feel like a whole woman. I needed to feel this myself first.

So, I am now on my way to true recovery. I am finally admitting I had breast cancer, and I need to find friends to speak to about having had it. This is real. This is scary. I am so tired of people thinking I will always be okay and I have nothing to worry about and talk about because I was able to beat breast cancer last year. SOMEONE PLEASE LISTEN TO ME, SOMEONE PLEASE HUG ME AND TELL ME YOU WILL LOVE ME. TREAT ME SPECIAL BECAUSE NOW YOU CAN APPRECIATE THAT AFTER MY BOUT WITH BREAST CANCER LAST YEAR I WAS SPARED AND BLESSED ENOUGH TO BE GIVEN MORE TIME.

Baby Steps

We as adults think that we can just have a thought and take off on
it
We forget the steps it takes to accomplish anything we want

Did we forget that we needed to learn to crawl and then learn
how to balance
before we could walk???

While I was on short-term leave for my hand surgery, I was able to get together with my girlfriends. After a month of going nuts sitting at home with only one good hand that was not my dominant one, I needed to reconnect with my friends. Work had consumed me once more, and I had lost touch with them again. I realized how much I need this connection. I have great friends and I missed them and should have them in my life. I realized that if work can consume me so much that I needed to sacrifice myself and disconnect from things that were important to me in life, then my career needed to take a real turn for the better so I could see changes on the horizon that needed to be made.

I went ahead and invited several of my friends over for dinner one evening, and to my surprise they all accepted and came. I didn't have to apologize for losing touch. When I extended the invitation, they accepted without a second thought. This felt so good to know it didn't matter to them that I had thrown myself back into my old ways. What mattered was that I kept resurfacing and wanted them in my life. We had so much fun that evening, and for me, it felt better to be around my girlfriends than any man I had in my life at the time. There is a wonderful bond with girlfriends and such a trust. I cannot let this go again. I have known Karen since junior high school. We were like sisters. She remembers things I can't even remember about my parents. I have known Debbie for over thirty years. We shared so many good times in the past. She is the absolute sweetest person you will ever meet in life. Claudia came over as well. Although I just met Claudia a couple of years ago when I moved into my community, she has become a very dear friend. We seem to have so much in common that there was an instant understanding and caring for one another. For myself, I need to make time to keep these women in my life. They mean so much to me.

I was able to go shopping with Merrill. I hadn't really done anything with Merrill since my breast cancer episode. She shared the day I went to the holistic doctor in New York and has always been there for me. How was I able to let so much time pass before we saw each other? Again, that old pattern just seemed to keep me away from the people I cared for the most. Merrill had lost a very close friend to cancer weeks before we spent some time together. This disease seems to be in our face always. It seems to come in different shapes and sizes, but the pain it causes is unspeakable at times. You have to wonder if this is how evil takes its shape in this world. Why does it attack the individuals it seems to choose? How does it choose? It doesn't quite seem to us to have any pattern. This is what makes it so devastating. You just can't head it off. All the money in the world won't stop it. When you are chosen by this disease, you have only God to turn to.

Once realizing I needed to get out of my present sales career, I decided I needed to do what I loved to do. What I believed in doing. What my gut was telling me to do. With that, I once again became a sales rep for Mannatech products. I believe in selling products you believe in. I have a contact name for one of our local hospitals and will try to introduce myself and the program that I am trying to initiate. This particular contact heads the holistic and all-natural department in this hospital. I believe it is the only area hospital that has a holistic department. I plan on leaving literature in as many places in Connecticut to introduce myself and the program that I feel has gotten me through some of the really tough times and has helped me mend and heal physically. I will give a percentage of the profits to a bank account I will entitle "Inner Circle." I am going to start a local chapter for women undergoing breast cancer treatment. I hope to get the supermarkets involved. My hope is that the supermarkets will donate nutritional food for those who cannot afford to get it for themselves. With profits I make from my Mannatech website, I will buy local women the supplement I took to keep me healing while undergoing my treatment. I still take this product every day faithfully. It just makes too much sense to me not to. I can't help but think how many more women would benefit from this supplement. I just have to get the message out there.

I have started to experiment with gourmet doggie treats. All organic ingredients from local businesses. Bailey loves the fact that he is my tester. He is stealing things more than ever in the house these days. I have been trying to train him with my treats. If he drops what he has in his mouth, I reward him with the treats. He got smart and figured it out. If he steals something and drops it, he will get treats whenever he wants them. I just can't win with this dog.

I took a ride to buy Bailey's dog food one day last week and in speaking to the owner, I let her know what I was doing with doggie treats. She was thrilled and said she wanted them and would give me some names of gourmet dog shops in Connecticut that would also be interested. As I said, if you believe in your product, it sells itself.

I will be visiting Andy, Merrill's husband, to help me set up a website for all of my products. A large percentage of the profits made will go to my Inner Circle bank account. I am hoping this will take off so that I can put more into my Inner Circle account and help more women undergoing breast cancer treatments. I am one person, but I know God will send me volunteers to help me when he feels it is time. Wouldn't it be wonderful if I could have this as my career? I would then be able to work with all the organic grocery stores in the area. Pick up fresh foods and drop them off to the local hospitals so that women could help themselves to nutritional foods and supplements. That's my dream. NO ONE WILL TAKE THIS FROM ME. I promised God I would get this off the ground, with his help of course. How wonderful would it be to have each state start an Inner Circle account and help their local women. I have a mission here and I need to get this started. It takes one person with enough faith in the process and in GOD to make miracles happen. It is my dream to see this through.

Special Visits - - - - - - - -
-- Special Moments

Have you ever felt as though you have met someone who reminds
you of someone you have lost?
Someone that was very dear to you?
Remember that lump that forms in your throat?

Is it because we so long to see them and long to be with them that
we find the similarities?
Is this consoling to us?

It's sad that we feel we have moved past the pain of the loss
But in one brief moment with someone sitting across from you or
someone just crossing the street
It will bring back someone you have lost and loved very much
It feels as though this cork explodes from this space deep inside
you
The space you have been holding all those memories that are
treasures
And you now are drowning in them
You can barely catch your breath

Do the people who have passed on feel this and take it as an
invitation to comfort us?
When you have those "memory moments" of a loved one who has
passed on
Did you ever wake up the next morning feeling as though they
had come to comfort you?

I truly believe they do

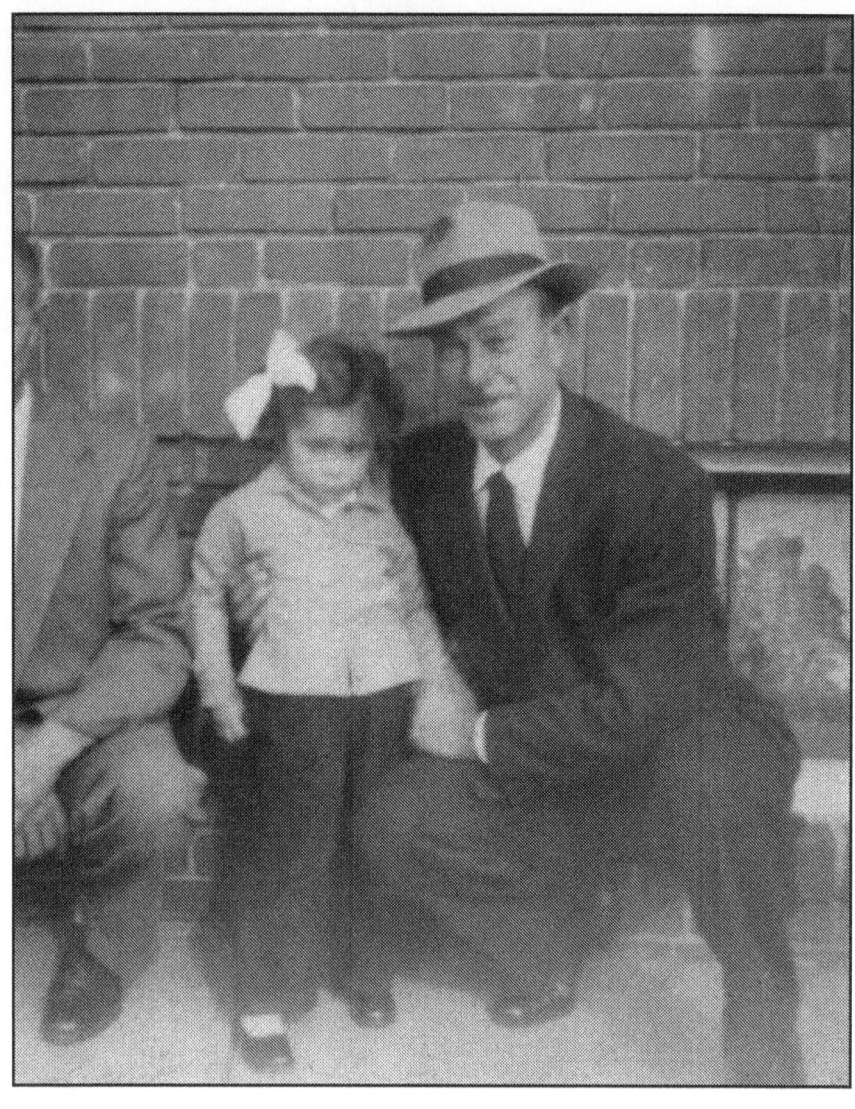

It was now June and it would be one year that I had been cancer free. My radiation treatments ended mid-June last year. My one-year cancer-free anniversary was creeping up on me. I had taken some MRIs back in April and they were negative. I had just done my mammogram and I was anxiously waiting for the results. I don't put these tests out of my head any longer. I wait to hear the results these days. They did check the x-rays while I was in the hospital taking the mammogram and told me it was okay to leave, as they could not see anything. There was a next step. A digital machine that the hospital had just purchased would check my x-rays, and I was waiting for the results from this "second opinion." I was sure everything was fine but wanted that call or letter verifying it.

I was so proud and grateful that I had been cancer free for one whole year now. I had a year under my belt. So, where were the people who were suppose to be grateful with me? Did they take my cancer-free time for granted? Was I expecting too much from everyone? Was there not anyone who was grateful I was okay after a year? Did anyone understand that there is no guarantee that the cancer would not surface again? Where were the people who loved me and wanted to celebrate the one-year mark with me?

It was like a curve ball that smacked me right between the eyes. I seemed to be the only one excited about my one-year anniversary. It seemed to me that after all I had gone through this past year— the stressful times at work, the breast cancer, my breaking it off with Rich and feeling so alone with all of this—I still made it. I WANTED A CELEBRATION!

No one seemed to understand this, and as usual I just silently hurt to myself. I didn't dare let anyone know what I was feeling.

Lord, they might understand and actually come through for me. I still needed emotional healing. This clearly stated, "Bruna, get some help."

I was feeling sorry for myself when I got a call from Claudia. She and her parents were going out to dinner that evening and she wanted me to come along. It was important to her that I meet her parents. They were elderly and her dad was so old-fashioned Italian. She wouldn't take no for an answer. I finally accepted, and as I hung up the phone, I realized that God had heard me. Here it was my celebration. I let Claudia know that this was going to be that celebration, as she'd saved me from going through this alone. How wonderful was this? I was so grateful.

Claudia and I met her parents at this quaint Italian restaurant. Claudia's dad was sitting directly across from me and I just got this pang in my heart. Her dad reminded me so much of my dad. He had the same mustache as my dad wore all of his life. You know the one—all the old movie stars back in the 40's had them. Her dad had my dad's charm and gestures, and the smile just got to me. It was that same twinkle in his smile. I had to swallow the tears that were trying to surface. Good Lord, how would I explain my getting this emotional over a dinner? Both of her parents were so gracious. I could not have picked a better one-year free celebration than this one. As we sat at the table enjoying our meal and conversation, they had no idea what this evening meant to me. I realized that evening why Claudia and I had become such good friends. We were raised the same way—we just had a different set of parents, but they were exactly the same. I felt I was sitting across from my parents, and this was such a gift to me. Claudia had no idea what she had given me that evening.

Once I got home from our dinner, I put on some comfortable clothes and could not hold back the tears any longer. I missed having my dad and mom around so much. You don't realize how you bury your feelings until something triggers them. Claudia's parents triggered my feelings for my parents and my pain for the loss of them. I wanted to sit across from my mom and dad so much. I have to believe that the ones who have passed on and crossed over do come to comfort us when we need them. When I got up the next morning after crying myself to sleep, I felt as though I had just left my dad. Could he have heard my invitation and visited me in my dreams? If you had asked me that morning, I would have had to tell you there was no doubt in my mind that I had spent time with my dad. I was comforted in a way only my dad could have comforted me.

A few weeks later I called Claudia to take a ride with me to look at a two-family house I was interested in as an investment. My older brother was meeting me at the house so he could give me his input on the investment. I wanted Claudia to meet my brother, as she knew how much my brother meant to me. My brother was a very successfully builder in town and I respected his opinion. We met the Realtors and did the walk-through. In the course of our conversation, Claudia noticed and later commented on the bond she felt and saw with my brother and me. I noticed as well, but explained to her I had to be careful with that, as it would surface once in a while and it took me back to our younger years. I knew he loved me, but he seemed to forget I was his sister, that I was alone, that I have a need for my family, and I suppose I expected him to be my brother when I needed a brother in my life now. Growing up, we'd had such a bond, and I always felt loved by my brother. Somehow he makes me feel insignificant these days. I feel I have been forgotten. A simple breakfast or lunch once in while would help us stay in touch. He makes time for others and I am his sister. I need him. I want him to make time for me. I need to feel his presence still in my life.

I need to step back and be grateful for my friends and what I do have in my life. My friends and my children are my family these days. This is my life today. I can't look back at yesterday. I need to accept and feel grateful for what I have, as so many have less than I do and some have nothing at all. I need to keep my heart open and enjoy the times I have with those I love. Like my brother Vince. He will always have a special place in my heart no matter what.

Curve Ball

Why is it when we think we are walking through life
and it's hard enough as it is
We get that curve ball?

I didn't seem to feel as though I was in the greatest space in life these days.

It was bad enough that I felt as though a tornado had come into my life and swooped me off onto a merry-go-round. I was dizzy and wanted to get off so bad. Kind of like when we were children and your mom put you on that object in the playground that made you dizzy as all hell? You know the one I mean. She would sit you on this plaything that was round and had bars that you held on to. It kind of looked like a huge wooden pie and the bars separated each piece of pie. You would be placed on one of the pieces and your mom would push the pie so that you would spin around and around. By the time mom let you off, you couldn't walk and you just wanted to vomit because you had become so dizzy. I never understood why adults thought we kids would enjoy this. The funny part is that once you got older, you would go to the same playground and actually be foolish enough to run in place with the pie and then jump on it so you could experience this same ridiculous dizziness as when your mom pushed you. Well, here I am an adult and I felt as though I had just gotten off this ride. I don't quite know how I got caught up in this whirlwind, but I was there and I just wanted to get off. I asked God's help in finding direction. Could this be the way he answers? It was time God needed to get my full attention once again.

I found myself desperately looking for jobs on the Internet while on my short-term leave for my hand surgery. Nothing seemed to catch my eye. I hated the thought of having to walk away from my present job, as I had given fourteen years to this company, and yet I hated the thought of going back. I had so many ideas in my head that could make me my own boss. I needed to finish my book to share with women who were single and going through breast cancer. I wanted to give them the message that there are many that go through this alone. I could have used a little book telling me it was okay to feel what I had during my breast cancer episode. I could find all of the knowledge and direction I needed. It was everywhere. What was missing was that little book that said "single with breast cancer."

I needed to start working on my website for the supplements that would help me start up my Inner Circle network and would allow me to help women going through the same journey as I had taken just one year ago myself. I needed to get the word out about my Inner Circle program. I needed to look for volunteers to help me get this off the ground. I needed to start baking my signature cookies and the gourmet doggie treats and get this piece going, as it would also help my Inner Circle program as well. How was I going to do all this and go back to work in just three weeks?

I woke up one morning after I decided I could do only one thing at a time. The first thing I needed to do was finish my book. I got up at 6 a.m. and after taking Bailey for his walk I made my coffee, sat at my computer, and started to finish my book. Within just a few hours, I received a call that just took me back some. It was about 10 a.m. I wasn't going to answer it, but it was Midstate Medical on the caller ID. My heart went to my throat. I just stared at the caller ID for a few seconds. I had just gone in for my mammogram a week ago. I knew they wouldn't be calling me to congratulate me on a good screening. I picked up the receiver and the woman on the other end of the phone proceeded to tell me that I needed to come in asap. They had found an area on my good breast that looked like a cluster of calcifications. This was the same call I'd received last year for my left breast. One year ago this month I'd finished radiation. I asked for an appointment to do the follow-up work and I was told to come in asap. I didn't need an appointment. I was told that they would be waiting for me and to get to radiology as soon as I could. I got off the phone and my whole body shook. I knew I couldn't do this again so soon. I just kept talking to God. While I showered, while I got dressed, while I put Bailey in his pen, and on my drive to the hospital, I kept saying, "I can't do this right now

God. Please not now. I'm not strong enough to fight right now. I need to get off of this whirlwind I'm in before I can do this again. I have no will to fight right now. Please help me." I drove into the hospital parking lot. I drove by the cancer patient parking and was pulling into a space. I looked at the sign. CANCER PATIENT PARKING. Hell, no way. I pulled out and found a regular parking space and said to myself, "No way are you getting me this time, you mother. And to think: I had just told God I didn't have any fight left in me.

I spent over three hours in radiology taking digital pictures, magnifying the pictures, and twisting my breast in ways I did not think were possible. All along I asked God to stay with me. God had already given me a sign. When I'd opened my car door to leave for the hospital, I had smelled cigarette smoke. This always made me feel my dad's presence. I don't quite know why, but when I smell cigarette smoke, I feel my dad around me. So I knew I had my dad and God with me. Finally after three hours the last sets of pictures were taken. My breast had been tortured. I looked down at the right breast and thought, "Wow, it did spring right back into shape." I cocked my head back and let it rest on the wall behind me. I had to wait what seemed like an eternity for the doctor to speak to me about what she found in the pictures taken of my "good breast." While I waited, I knew I had God and I had my dad with me. I closed my eyes and felt this warm white light around me. I just basked in it as if I were sitting at the beach with the sun beating warmly on me. The doctor knocked on my door and all I could say was, "Yes?" I felt my heart go right to my throat. The door opened, the doctor looked at me, and I was prepared. "We can't find anything" is all the doctor had to say to me. "You're okay to leave. We're done. See you next year." I looked at her and my first thought was, "What do you mean you can't find anything? Where did the cluster go? Did it dissolve?" I had been shown the mammo x-rays with the light area and now they were nowhere to be found? No good explanation was given to me other than it may have been something else. Somehow I know God had his hand in this. How could the doctor possibly know the relationship I had with God, and how could she possibly know that God and my dad were with me through this whole procedure?

When I got to my car, I called my girlfriend in New Jersey, Judith—my very spiritual and great friend. Judith is the definition of the saying that God gives us tools and sends angels to help us and guide us to show us the way. Judith was my first thought and she was my first call. "Hi Judith. I'm just leaving the hospital and I am a miracle. Call me when you get the chance. I want to share this with you. Only you can know how I feel right now and only you can understand how full of love and gratitude I am right now."

She called within five minutes.

Grateful Grateful Grateful

A very dear friend of mine has introduced me to a song recently
Grateful by Hezekiah Walker

I now start my days by playing this song
I want to begin every day with gratefulness

God has given me so much to be grateful for
I have been given God's work to do
I am reminded every day of my life by starting my day with
gratitude.

I pray for the strength to accomplish what is meant for me in this
lifetime
I will then leave my signature

One more person through God and gratitude will complete her
role while walking on this mortal path with spirit

Grateful

Judith was my silent strength through my breast cancer experience and thereafter. She seemed to become my minister. There was no negative in my life, as Judith would not have it. If I started to sink into a victim role, it was Judith who would spiritually pick me up. Oh, don't get me wrong, she gave me a kick in the ass many times when I needed it. It did not matter that I was going through surgery or radiation or riding on an emotional roller coaster. Judith was the word of God. It seemed as though God needed to find an earthly soul to speak to me. I was having such a hard time understanding God speaking to me that I truly believe he sent me Judith. One would have to listen to Judith. She is a powerful, intelligent, successful, spiritual, and very proud "woman of color," as Judith would say. She has the loveliest skin. Judith is one of those individuals that you would have to meet to understand her beauty inside and out. She is a true example that there are no words to describe............ Judith.

I met Judith several years ago. She was hired as my manager and was not the usual internal hire. She came from the "outside," and it was so refreshing to have her. The first trip she made to my office in Connecticut was an instant bond. Judith worked out of our NYC office, so I wasn't able to have the honor of her presence every day. Unprofessionally I gave her a hug when I met her, rather than the usual handshake. It was instinct on my part, and I felt comfortable doing so. After I hugged her, I looked at her and said, "I feel as though I know you already." Little did I know that day that we would find ourselves talking and realize we were both children of God. Due to reorganization in our company, Judith was my manager for only a brief few months. We stayed in touch always. When Judith found out I had breast cancer, our calls seemed to be on a daily basis. If not daily, we didn't let many days go by without speaking or text messaging one another. Judith kept me positive every day. She was so instrumental in my getting through my ordeal spiritually. Judith made me realize that you need only one person of God in your life to help you through and keep you in tune to who you are and who is always there for you. God. He never fails us. You ask and he will deliver.

Unfortunately Judith lives in New Jersey and I live in Connecticut, so we didn't get to see much of each other. Judith was there for me when I went back to work after my breast cancer ordeal. It worked out for me that she worked for the same division in our organization as I did. This would allow her to understand what I was going through. She kept me encouraged. Judith and I both realized within six months upon my returning to work after breast cancer surgery and radiation that this sales team and I were not going to work out. I stuck out like a sore thumb and just could not fit into this group. I was not compromising myself, and the writing was on the wall for me.

Judith did not visit Connecticut often, so when I received a call from her recently and she surprised me with the news that she would be coming to Connecticut on business and would be able to stay overnight, I was thrilled. I couldn't wait to see her. We made plans that once Judith arrived in Connecticut and she finished up with all of her meetings planned for her that day, she would call me and I would meet her at the hotel. When I arrived, we took some time to sit and chat. We finally got hungry and decided on an Italian bistro in town. Judith was in the mood for "good" Italian food and we were off. Judith shared her good news with me. She had found a position outside of our company that she was ecstatic about. I was so happy for her good fortune. God had helped her out and we decided I was next. We both knew I would not be able to stay with this company very long. Where I ended up was not clear, but God had his plan for me as well. It was tough saying goodbye to her at the end of the evening. Even though we spoke daily, it was just not the same. It was so good to sit across the table from Judith at the restaurant as we talked and laughed. I would give anything to have her live close by so that I could pick up the phone and say, "Come over for a glass of wine and let's talk." Her presence is so powerful that you feel blessed to have her in your life. The night did end, and we did say goodbye.

Judith was my first call from the hospital when I had my "scare" this go-around with my "good breast." We seemed to be playing phone tag on my drive home from the hospital. Thinking I might have cancer in my good breast was disturbing, so I took the drive home to get myself together. I felt so grateful it was a false alarm. I would call Judith back when I got home so that I could share what I was feeling with her with no distractions. When I pulled into my driveway, I took a seat on the side of my house next to the butterfly bush. My favorite spot. I had small white butterflies dancing all around me. Some looked like they had partners and shared them with others. This was the butterfly bush I had waited at for my spicebush swallowtail to come back to visit me last year. I sat by the bush in the sun talking to Judith. After I shared the experience I had just gone through at Midstate Hospital, she kept repeating over and over again, "You need to listen to this song. It's called "Grateful." If she said it once, she said it a hundred times. I promised I would get it asap. I didn't pick it up until a few days later. I couldn't wait to get the wrapper off and pop it into my CD player. Judith had gone on and on about it. I finally got my chance to listen to "Grateful." I had it blaring, the windows down, the sun beating on me through my sun roof, and I just swelled up. There it was in music, My Testimony. My chest was just ready to burst. I felt so much love and gratitude that I didn't know how I could contain all of this.

That day was the first day of summer. That evening I grabbed Bailey and headed out to the ocean. We had just had a huge thunderstorm, but I didn't care. That didn't hold me back, as I needed to meet God at our ocean and thank him personally. The ocean was always our meeting place. God was always there waiting for me. When Bailey and I drove by the ocean to find a good spot to park the car, the sun was shining and it was absolutely beautiful. I noticed that Bailey loved the ocean just as much as I did. Before we left, I found a huge piece of driftwood to rest on. I had tired Bailey out as we ran along the ocean on the beach. Most of the time, he was running in the ocean shallows and I was trying to stay on shore. He sat by me and we both focused on the sun setting over the ocean. "Hey Bailey," I said. "This is where I was when I found out you were going to belong to me. Out of over a hundred calls, she picked me to own you." I gave him a hug and he licked my hand.

This was God's plan. I knew it then. I finally got what Bailey was all about in my life. All Bailey had put me through, breaking me down to tears, challenging me, driving me nuts and right to the edge. I'd needed someone to bring me to that point through this ordeal or I might never have cried, I might never have coughed up the pain and grief I had been holding on to. He had the spirit I needed in my life at this time. I could not have benefited from any other spirit than his in this past year.

All that Bailey had put me through. His love, his trust, his loyalty, and his constantly letting me know I was the most important thing to him. It wasn't going to matter what I looked like, how bad or good things got, or where I ended up in life. As long as I was in his life, he was going to be the happiest dog in the world. I mattered. I was the most important thing to Bailey, and no one could deny this.

Yep, Bailey my buddy and I sat there at the beach that evening, the first day of summer watching the sun go down. Thank you God and know that I am grateful every day of my life for all you have given me. Please give me the strength to do your work as you have a plan for me. As crazy as it may seem to anyone else............... Let's do it ....together.

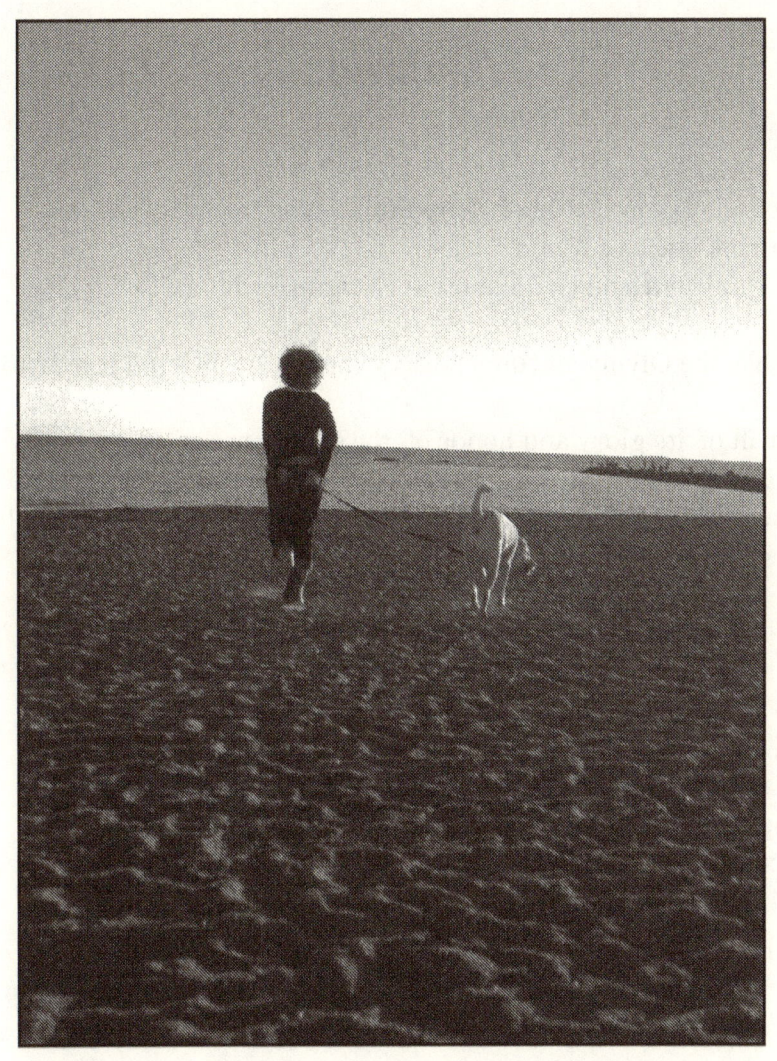

Friends

For all of you that have shared this experience with me
I thank you as a friend
For only a friend could know such intimacy of me

I, like the Olympian runner, carry the torch and hand it over to
you
In all of its glory and honor of the experience of this journey
God has chosen to send me out on
Carry this torch to its final destination with thankfulness of all
the knowledge we have gained

The person we have become because of this journey
The strength and endurance in life we have shown that we could
have not demonstrated without this experience

Take this into the rest of your life and become what you were
meant to be
Experience all God has wanted for you
Make this a journey without longing

Be the example we were destined to be
And be proud to have been one of the chosen ones

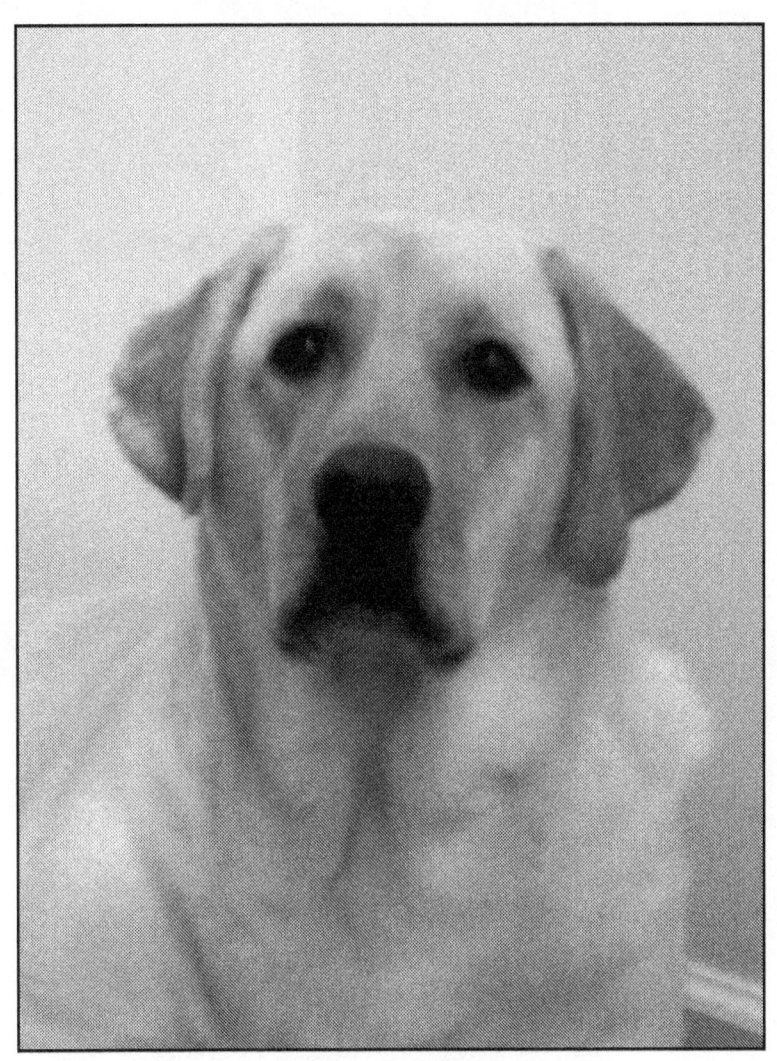

Precious